CARDIOLOGY RESEARCH AND CLINICAL DEVELOPMENTS

# 24 HOUR HEART RATE VARIABILITY ANALYSIS (HRV) IN CHILDHOOD

## PROGNOSTIC SIGNIFICANCE, RISK FACTORS AND CLINICAL APPLICATIONS

## "WHAT CHILDREN'S HEARTS WANT TO TELL"

# CARDIOLOGY RESEARCH AND CLINICAL DEVELOPMENTS

Additional books in this series can be found on Nova's website under the Series tab.

Additional e-books in this series can be found on Nova's website under the e-book tab.

CARDIOLOGY RESEARCH AND CLINICAL DEVELOPMENTS

# 24 HOUR HEART RATE VARIABILITY ANALYSIS (HRV) IN CHILDHOOD

## PROGNOSTIC SIGNIFICANCE, RISK FACTORS AND CLINICAL APPLICATIONS

## "WHAT CHILDREN'S HEARTS WANT TO TELL"

REINER BUCHHORN, M.D.

NOVA BIOMEDICAL

*New York*

**Library of Congress Cataloging-in-Publication Data**

ISBN: 978-1-63463-825-8

Library of Congress Control Number: 2014959223

*Published by Nova Science Publishers, Inc. † New York*

# Contents


| | | |
|---|---|---|
| **Preface** | | **vii** |
| **Abbreviations** | | **ix** |
| **Chapter 1** | Methods | **1** |
| **Chapter 2** | HRV and New Morbidity in Childhood | **13** |
| **Chapter 3** | The Impact of Body Mass Index, Caloric Intake and Omega-3-Fatty Acids on HRV | **21** |
| **Chapter 4** | HRV and Mental Health | **45** |
| **Chapter 5** | Sports and HRV | **51** |
| **Chapter 6** | HRV in Children with Heart Disease | **55** |
| **Chapter 7** | HRV and Growth | **73** |
| **Chapter 8** | Effects of Pharmacotherapy on HRV | **77** |
| **Chapter 9** | Autonomic Programming | **93** |
| **Chapter 10** | HRV and Death | **99** |
| **Conclusion** | | **105** |
| **References** | | **107** |
| **Index** | | **121** |

# Preface

The project "What Children's Hearts Want to Tell" is a 20 year old project of the author to explain that frequent diseases in childhood are related to regulation disorder of the autonomic nervous system. I started the project in 1996 with the introduction of beta-blocker therapy for heart failure in infants with heart disease. In my recent review article titled "The long way to a successful medical therapy of heart failure with beta-blockers in children with heart disease" together with some colleagues we were able to confirm the hypothesis that this longtime unpopular therapy may save many children's lives.

Having observed the increase in mental disease in childhood, I shifted the focus in 2005 to the "New Morbidity in Childhood". This publication now presents a comprehensive model how autonomic dysfunction may cause cognitive disorders, growth failure, heart failure as well as frequent mental diseases that are not well understood today such as fatigue- and pain syndromes. This new understanding will help us to improve the therapy.

Last but not least this model can be a road map to understand the new morbidities in children and to effectively treat the causes of frequent diseases like obesity and attention deficit disorder. And by effectively treating these conditions in children's lives we come back to the core of this model and may be able to improve the cardiovascular prognosis for adult life, which is the main cause of human mortality.

At a time when the value of a medical innovation depends on its economic value and despite the national recognition of my work, it proved impossible to gain support for further research from university institutions. As a result, in 2005 I continued my research while head of a small pediatric department in the rural part of southern Germany. Here, far away from academic competition, I found a group of professionals committed to understanding children's biology. Without financial support, we have systematically performed nearly 1000 Holter ECG measurements to understand children's autonomic nervous system. I thank the superb technical assistance of my colleagues Cornelia Weiss, Helga Zimmermann, Julia Fischer and Karl-Heinz Stump. In addition, I thank my colleagues Dr. Christian Willaschek, Dr. Lara Mänhardt, Dr. Sonja Dippacher, Dr. Christian Müller, Dr. Susanne Feeg, Hanna Lang and Dr. Tünde Kertess-Szlaninka who have helped me to publish our data - the most problematic but perhaps the most important task for a passionate researcher. This book also includes doctors' theses from Sebastian Meint (HRV and growth), Marie-Sophie Richwalski (Sports) and Franziska Hauk (HRV and nutrition). In the near future further students will analyze our data from 150 children treated with psycho-stimulants, 80 children with diabetes mellitus and 50 obese children with metabolic syndrome. This data will be included in future revisions of this book.

30.10.2014

Prof. Dr. med. Reiner Buchhorn
Department of Pediatrics
Caritas Krankenhaus Bad Mergentheim
Uhlandstr. 7
97980 Bad Mergentheim, Germany
e-mail: reiner.buchhorn@ckbm.de
Tel.: 00497931582301
Fax.: 00497931582390

# Abbreviations

| | |
|---|---|
| ADHD | Attention Deficit Hyperactivity Disorder |
| BMI | Body Mass Index |
| BNP | Brain Natriuretic Peptide |
| BPA | Bisphenol A |
| CGD | Constitutional Growth Delay |
| CHD | Congenital Heart Defect |
| FFA | Fast Fourier Analysis |
| GHD | Growth Hormone Deficiency |
| GUCH | Grown up with Congenital Heart Defect |
| HC | Healthy Control |
| HF | High Frequency Power |
| HRV | Heart Rate Variability |
| ICT | Information and Communication Ttechnology |
| LF | Low Frequency Power |
| MPD | Methylphenidate |
| MRI | Magnetic Resonance Imaging |
| NGS | Naso Gastric tube feeding |
| NICE | National Institute for Health and Care Excellence |
| PM | Particulate Matter |
| PN | Parenteral Nutrition |
| pNN50/sNN50 | Absolute number (sNN50) or number of pairs of adjacent NN intervals differing by more than 50ms divided by the total number of all NN intervals (pNN50) |
| PVC | Premature Ventricular Contractions |
| rMSSD | Square root of the arithmetic mean of the |

| | |
|---|---|
| | squared deviation of successive normal RR intervals |
| SDNN | Standard deviation of all normal RR intervals in a time frame |
| SGA | Small for Gestational Age |
| TP | Total Power |
| VLF | Very Low Frequency Power |

*Chapter 1*

# Methods

## 1.1. Methodical Basics

Fundamental to all HRV data analysis is a group of successive normal RR intervals in sinus rhythm (so-called NN intervals in comparison to RR intervals in cardiac arrhythmia) in a defined period of time in minutes (so called short-term HRV) or in 24 hours (so-called long-term HRV) (1996). The Time Domain Analysis is done by the processing of the data with simple statistical methods. For didactic reasons in this study we focus on the statistical analysis of the following 4 parameters, which are briefly outlined below:

1) *Heart rate:* The easiest but very important HRV parameter is the average sinus rhythm heart rate, since all other parameters are significantly affected by the heart rate.
2) *SDNN:* Standard deviation of all normal RR intervals in a time frame. This global HRV parameter represents the overall variability of the autonomic nervous system.
3) *rMSSD: Square* root of the arithmetic mean of the squared deviation of successive normal RR intervals in a time frame. This parameter is mainly influenced by the parasympathetic nervous system.
4) *sNN50/pNN50:* Absolute number (sNN50) or number of pairs of adjacent NN intervals differing by more than 50ms divided by the total number of all NN intervals (pNN50). This parameter is mainly influenced by the parasympathetic nervous system.

The technical background of the so-called Frequency Domain Analysis is the Fast Fourier Analysis of the consecutive NN intervals. If the whole variability is represented as the Total Power in time elapsed, we can produce the 3 graphs of 3 adolescents demonstrated in Figure 1.1. These "prime graphs" of the HRV are evocative of an EEG, so that I would like to call them the EEG of our autonomic network. This was initially described by Claude Bernard and more recently by Julian Thayer (Thayer & Lane, 2009). I would like to emphasize, that by the HRV analysis we don't analyze the heart, but the autonomic regulation centers of our brain, especially the limbic system and the hypothalamus. Keeping this in mind, the HRV analysis provides us with a unique insight into our emotional regulatory system, which we otherwise could only detect in functional magnetic resonance imaging (MRI) examinations (Thayer et al., 2012). The major advantage especially for the pediatric population is the possibility to measure the HRV of the young patients unnoticed, under real life conditions with little costs and without the artificial and expensive conditions of an MRI.

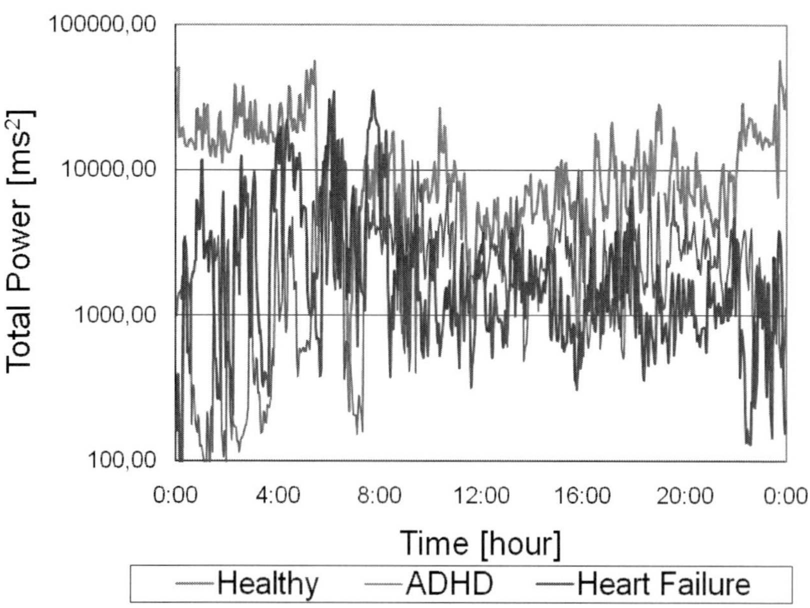


Figure 1.1. Total (HRV) Power of three 16 years old adolescents: 1) Attention Deficit Disorder 2) severe Heart Failure 3) Healthy Control.

## 1.2. Comparison of Methods by Case Reports

As introduction to the topic I present the HRV parameters of three 16 years old adolescents by different methods (Figure 1.1, 1.2 and 1.3). These show the comparison of a healthy control patient with an ideal autonomic regulatory system with 2 patients with pathologically reduced HRV; one with attention deficit hyperactivity disorder (ADHD) under treatment with Methylphenidate and a second with severe heart failure due to dilated cardiomyopathy.

At first glance, the 24 hours Total Power in Figure 1.1 shows different values for the 3 adolescents at night while showing big overlaps during daytime. The differences are so profound that the y-axis had to be changed into a logarithmic scale. We recently described this missing vagal activity at night time in systematic reviews of adolescents with ADHD (Buchhorn et al., 2012a) and the changes in this case are much more striking than in a boy of the same age with severe heart failure. The reduced HRV in heart failure has already been described numerous times and has prognostic value.

The 24 hours mean value of the Time Domain Analysis in Figure 1.2 presents clearly the loss of the HRV in the boys with ADHD and heart failure. However the mean heart rate is within the average range for their age.

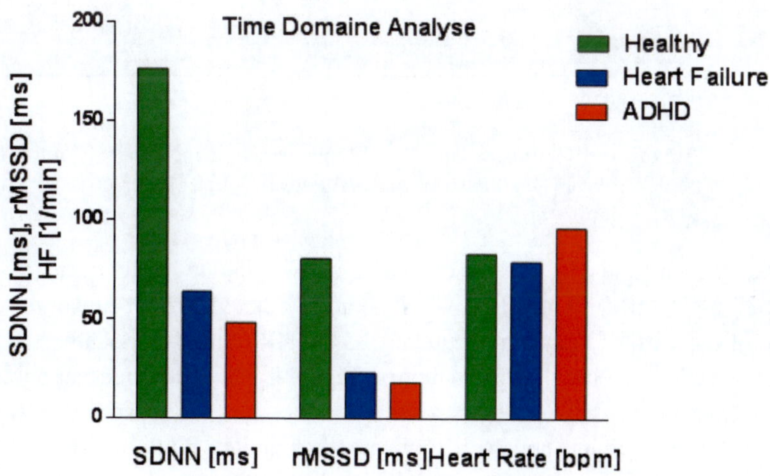


Figure 1.2. Time Domain Analysis of three 16 years old adolescents with attention deficit disorder and severe heart failure compared to a healthy proband.

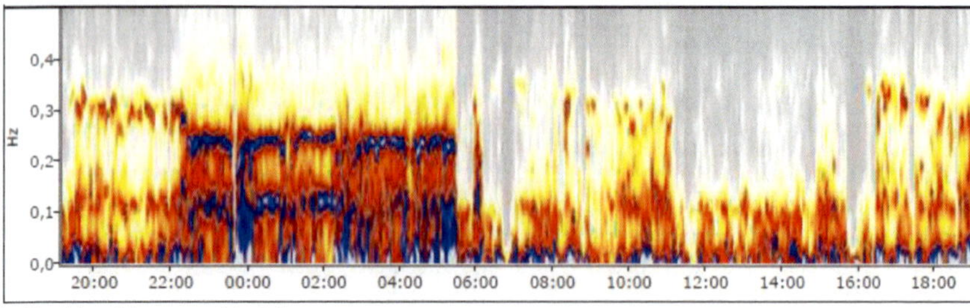


1: Healthy 16 years old girl

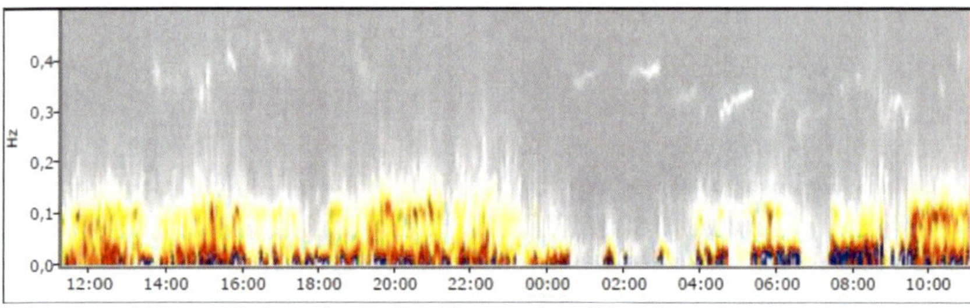


2: 16 years old boy with Attention Deficit Hyperactivity Disorder

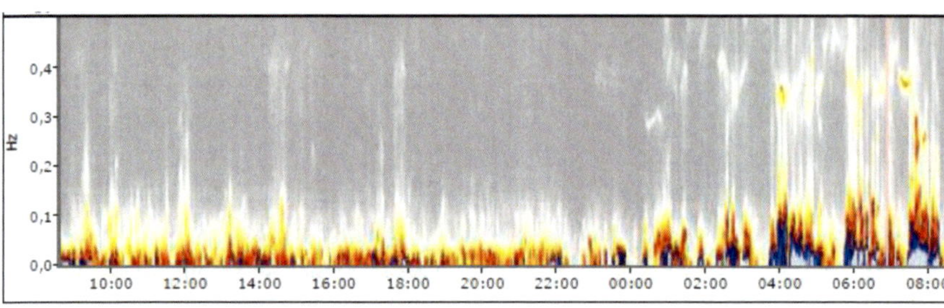


3: 16 years old boy with severe heart failure

Figure 1.3. "Fire of Life" ™ illustration of the Frequency Domaine Analysis of three 16 years old adolescents: 1) Healthy Control 2) Attention Deficit Hyperactivity Disorder 3) Heart Failure.

Yet the diverse HRV is also clearly shown in the "Fire of Life" ™ illustration (SCHILLERmedilog, Wiesbaden, Germany), which illustrates the power of the various ranges in frequency of the HRV in a color scheme (from grey, via yellow, to blue) over 24 hours (Figure 1.3). The perfect autonomic regulation of the healthy control is reflected in the high (blue) activity between 0,1 and 0,3 Hz (which equals 6 to18 breaths/minute) at night time, which represents the respiratory sinus arrhythmia as an expression of the vagal activity at night. Even during daytime, e.g. while attending art classes between 10 and 11 am and after school at 4 pm we can see vagal stimulation as a sign of mental recovery while still being awake. During Math and Latin classes between 11am and 1pm we can see a strong 0.1 Hz band as a sign of concentration. While doing exercise by cycling to and from school around 7.30am and 3.30pm vagal activity is almost completely suppressed. These modulations which are circadian and adjusted to the autonomic requirements are not evident in the two ill boys. The two boys with ADHD and severe heart failure display no HRV above 0,1 Hz and while asleep, show a complete loss of their HRV.

## 1.3. Trend of HRV within a Lifetime

The standard HRV values for children were published in 1997 by Massin (Massin & von Bernuth, 1997). Standard values for adults were published in 2010 for the United States (Zulfiqar et al., 2010c) and in 2005 for German patients by H. Bonnemeier (Bonnemeier et al., 2003b). During the course of life these standard values show most importantly 2 trends:

1) Figure 1.4 illustrates the regression curves of global HRV (SDNN) and the vagal parameter rMSSD during the course of the life of a healthy human being from birth to 80 years of age. The striking increase of vagal activity from birth up to the age of 15 years is typical of healthy children. There is a decline of HRV and vagal activity with age in adults with very similar data in the United States (Zulfiqar et al., 2010b) and Germany (Bonnemeier et al., 2003a).
2) These age dependant changes go along with different circadian rhythms as shown in Figure 1.5.

In our own evaluation of standard values 2012 we identified a significant vagal shift in childhood in comparison to the historical normal values measured in 1997, while still having the same heart rate and global HRV in 157 children at the age of birth to 16 years (De Bock et al., 2013).

A main methodological problem of HRV analysis is contradictory normal values of published data for healthy control groups. For example there is a wide range of rMSSD values for healthy adolescents between 47 +/- 25 ms and 89 +/- 45 ms in four different publications from Turkey. These differences are probably caused by different Holter ECG systems and inadequately defined control groups.

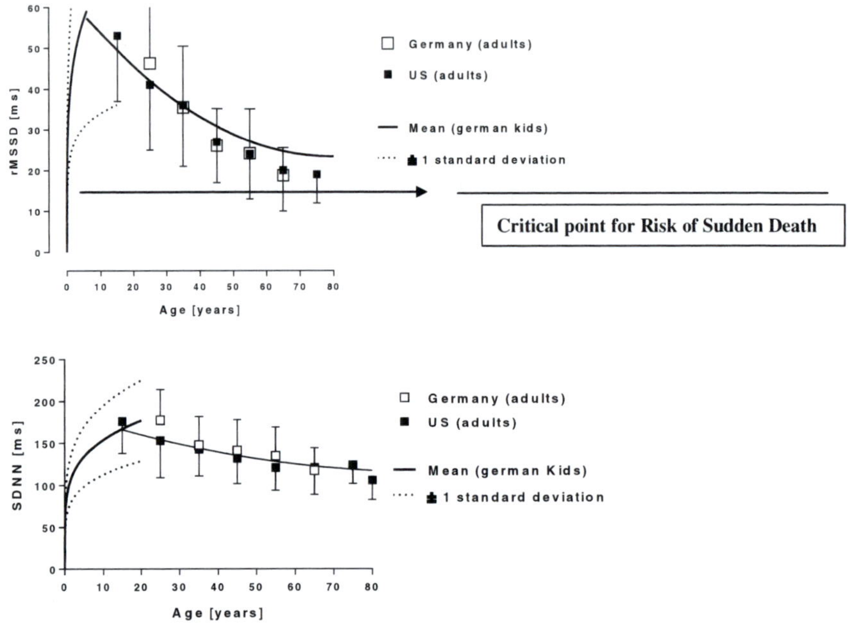


Figure 1.4. Trend of HRV within a lifetime. Interestingly normal values in the classical risk groups of sudden (unexpected) death below 1 year and over 60 years lying under the critical point of 15ms, as described in adults with sudden death.

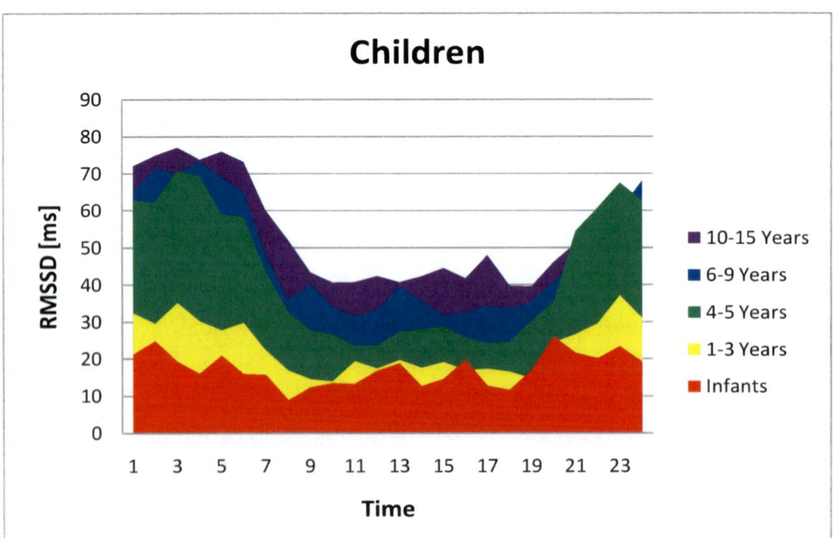

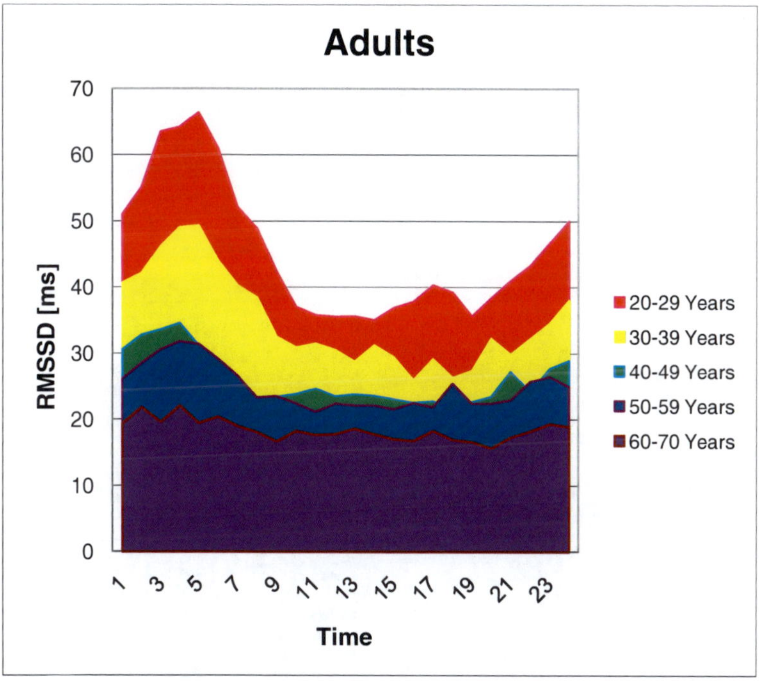


Figure 1.5. Circadian Vagus Activity indicated by rMSSD in different age groups.

## 1.4. Comparison of Different Measuring Systems for HRV Analysis

The standard values of 1997 were measured with the Medilog® equipment by the Oxford Company. Our measurements have been carried out using the 24 hours ECG Pathfinder® by the Reynolds Medical Systems (today SpaceLab Healthcare). Since diverse algorithms for analysis have been used to date by the different companies, we did simultaneous evaluations on 22 patients with the Pathfinder® and the succession model Medilog Darwin® by the Schiller Company. The best correlation with the Medilog ® system we achieved using the additional HRVTool® in the Time Domain Analysis (Figure 1.6). The correlation of the Frequency Domain Analysis was too unreliable to be used for our HRV score.

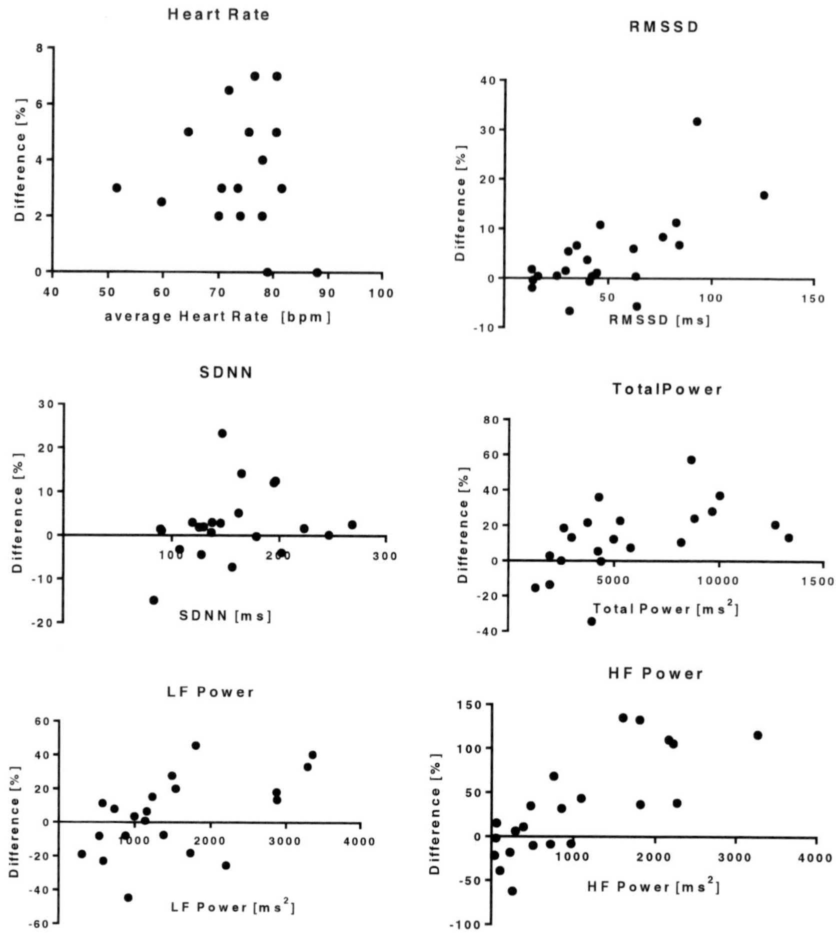


Figure 1.6. Bland-Altman Plots (Difference versus Average) of different HRV parameters measured with Medilog® or Pathfinder®.

## 1.5. HRV Score

It is not possible to compare HRV data between different age groups due to the age dependency of normal HRV values. Furthermore it is not possible to compare longitudinal HRV data in childhood. To overcome these important limitations of HRV analysis I introduced a HRV score that indicates the individual global autonomic balance related to the age specific normal values. Our own values from healthy children in combination with the standard values published in 2005 by H. Bonnemeier for German adults (measured with the same equipment) enabled us to quote mean values including standard deviations for the ages from birth to 70 years (Table 1.1).

**Table 1.1. HRV Score based upon mean and one standard deviation for the ages from birth to 70 years**

| Children | | Mean ± 1 standard deviation (Time Domain Analysis) | | | | Day to Night Ratio | |
|---|---|---|---|---|---|---|---|
| Heart Rate | Age | - 1 SD | Mean | +1 SD | | [%] | |
| | 0-1 | 119 | 128 | 137 | | | higher=1 |
| | >1-3 | 111 | 118 | 125 | | < 10 | Ratio=1 |
| | >3-6 | 89 | 98 | 107 | | <15 | lower= -1 |
| | >6-10 | 83 | 90 | 97 | | <15 | |
| | >10-16 | 73 | 81 | 90 | | <15 | |
| SDNN | 0-1 | 62 | 72 | 82 | | | lower=2 |
| (Global HRV) | >1-3 | 66 | 82 | 99 | | | higher= -1 |
| | >3-6 | 89 | 115 | 132 | | | |
| | >6-10 | 116 | 141 | 165 | | | |
| | >10-16 | 128 | 173 | 218 | | | |
| rMSSD | 0-1 | 13 | 18 | 22 | | | lower=1 |
| (Vagal) | >1-3 | 16 | 21 | 26 | | <20 | Ratio=1 |
| | >3-6 | 27 | 41 | 55 | | <30 | higher = -1 |
| | >6-10 | 32 | 46 | 60 | | <30 | |
| | >10-16 | 35 | 52 | 70 | | <15 | |
| Adults | | 24 hour Mean (Time Domain Analysis) | | | | Day to Night Ratio | |
| Heart Rate | Age | - 1SD Men | + 1SD | - 1SD Women | +1SD | [%] | |
| | 20-29 | 65 | 81 | 69 | 88 | <15 | higher=1 |
| | 30-39 | 69 | 84 | 73 | 89 | <12 | Ratio=1 |
| | 40-49 | 69 | 84 | 73 | 94 | <10 | lower= -1 |
| | 50-59 | 66 | 79 | 71 | 87 | <10 | |
| | 60-69 | 66 | 82 | 69 | 87 | <10 | |
| SDNN | 20-29 | 146 | 218 | 138 | 210 | | lower=2 |
| | 30-39 | 122 | 188 | 112 | 178 | | higher=-1 |
| | 40-49 | 112 | 184 | 84 | 156 | | |
| | 50-59 | 106 | 174 | 101 | 149 | | |
| | 60-69 | 94 | 146 | 74 | 126 | | |
| rMSSD | 20-29 | 33 | 69 | 22 | 58 | < 20 | lower=1 |
| | 30-39 | 21 | 51 | 20 | 50 | <15 | Ratio=1 |
| | 40-49 | 20 | 38 | 17 | 35 | <10 | higher = -1 |
| | 50-59 | 15 | 35 | 14 | 34 | <10 | |
| | 60-69 | 13 | 25 | 13 | 25 | 0 | |

**Table 1.2. Interpretation of the HRV Score**

| HRV Score | Interpretation |
|---|---|
| (-2) - (-3) | Vagotone State |
| (-1) - 1 | Normal Value |
| 2 - 3 | Autonomic Dysfunction 1° |
| 4 - 6 | Autonomic Dysfunction 2° |

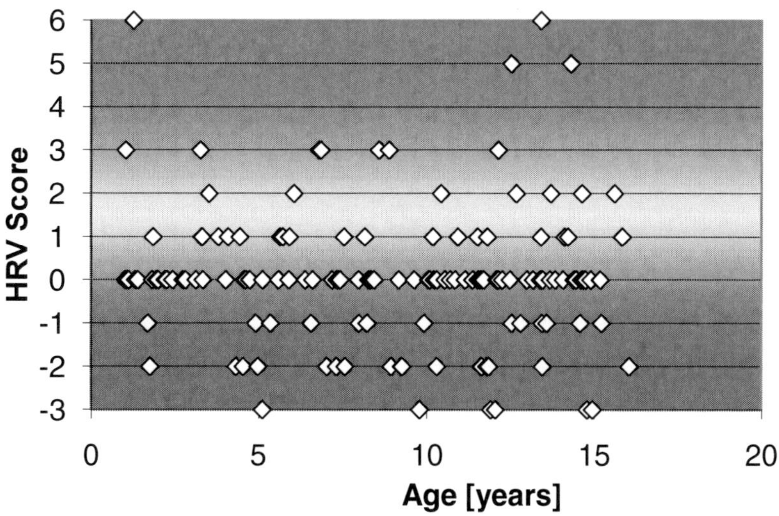


Figure 1.7. Illustration of 157 healthy children with the HRV Score.

For the HRV score we rated the deviation of each of the 3 time domain parameters: heart rate, SDNN and rMSSD and their day/night ratio into a scoring system (Table 1.2). Due to the unstable day/night rhythms in early infancy we were unable to quote any circadian values for the parameter SDNN. In this case we used a scoring system with 2 scores per parameter. The maximum possible score for the 3 parameters (heart rate, SDNN and rMSSD) is a HRV score of 6. An elevated HRV will be marked negative for each parameter, so that the minimum score is (-)3. With the calculated score we can do an evaluation as demonstrated in Table 1.2. The rainbow color scheme is used for all the graphs (red/yellow = reduced HRV, green = normal range, blue = elevated HRV). Figure 1.7 shows the autonomic regulation of 157 healthy children pictured as HRV score. It demonstrates the normally distributed values with 4 spikes into the red zone in severe autonomic dysfunctions in the age group from birth to 16 years. Since the inclusion criteria eliminated organic and obvious psychiatric diseases, these 4 patients seem to have an unapparent dysregulation of their autonomic nervous system. Patients with a so-called vagotone state (HRV score -2/-3) could for example represent athletes.

## 1.6. Clinical Applications

Our self-designed HRV score have been used for more than 1000 children with various somatic and psychosomatic illnesses (Figure 1.8). So at first glance autonomic dysfunction in a variety of diseases and their severity can be recognized. For the first time it's possible to illustrate the changes of the autonomic nervous system in the long-term and to use it to control the successful therapy, because age dependent alterations of the HRV parameter can be compensated by validation with age related standard values.

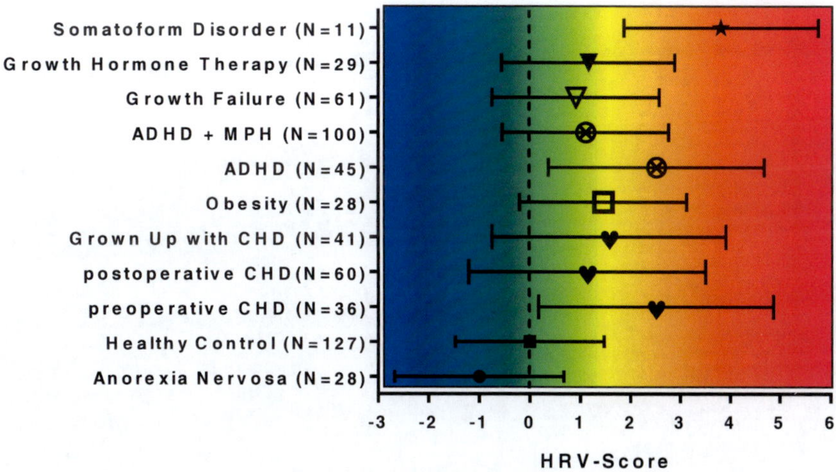


Figure 1.8. Autonomic regulation of 566 children with various somatic and psychosomatic illnesses illustrated with the HRV Score.

*Chapter 2*

# HRV and New Morbidity in Childhood

Why are mental and eating disorders – the so called new morbidity in childhood - becoming more and more common? This question haunts us pediatricians as well as many teachers and the affected parents.

## 2.1. Epidemiologic Data

Epidemiologic data, such as the number of admitted children and adolescents with psychiatric disorders as reported by the Statistics Center of Baden Wuerttemberg, Germany, or the prescriptions of the psycho-active drug Methylphenidate (MPH) through the public health system show that this is not only a subjective impression (Figure 2.1). There is comparable data in USA showing an increase of ADHD cases by 21.8% between the years of 2007 and 2010. Recently the US Center of Disease Control estimated a 12 month prevalence of any mental disorder for children between 8 and 15 years to be 13.1%. Leading diagnosis are attention deficit disorder (8.6%), mood disorders (3.7%), major depression (2.1%) and conduct disorders (2.1%). In this analysis the prevalence of eating disorders with 0.1% seems to be low, however, 17% of children suffer from obesity. This so called "New Morbidity in Childhood" is accompanied by increasing costs for mental health and cardiovascular disease in all age groups. The global cost of mental health is estimated to cost US$6 trillion by 2030, increasing from US$2.5 trillion in 2010, while cardiovascular disease is estimated to cost US$ 1.04 trillion by 2030 (rising from US$ 863 billion in 2010) (Bloom et al., 2011). Critically, there is increasing recognition that these disorders are related: depression is independently associated with cardiovascular morbidity and mortality, and is common among patients with cardiovascular disease (Carney and Freedland, 2009; Lichtman et al., 2008). All these diseases are related to autonomic dysfunction with a high impact on prognosis (Thayer & Lane, 2007). Recently we could demonstrate a decrease of vagal activity in healthy children and speculate that insufficient vagal maturation may be a reason for an increasing prevalence of mental and cardiovascular disease.

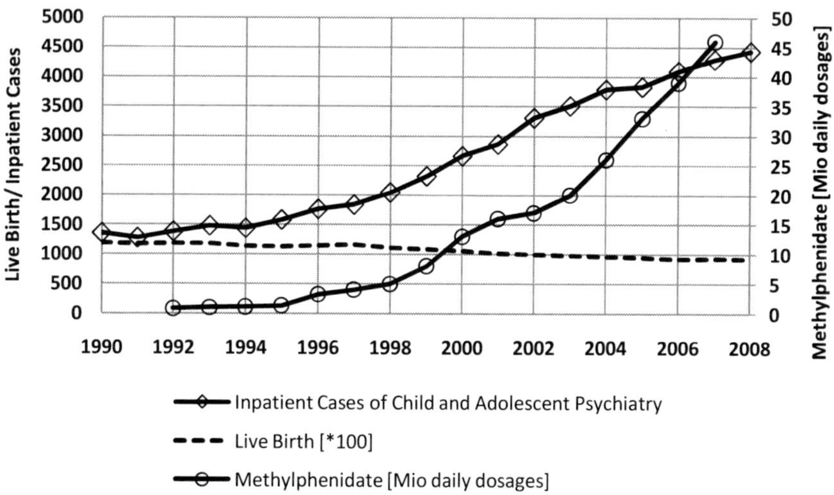


Figure 2.1. Inpatient cases of child and adolescent psychiatry and live births according to the data of the Statistics Center of Baden Württemberg, Germany. Number of daily methylphenidate dosages (insurance data from Germany).

## 2.2. Choice of an Appropriate Pathophysiologic Model

Why do experts hesitate to further investigate the causes of this increase in pediatric psychiatric cases in our modern industrialized society? Probably this is mainly a methodological problem of most sociological studies. The "epidemic" of pediatric psychiatric disorders coincides with current demographic change and globalization. This implies that many influencing factors like changing family constellations, media consumption or nutrition have simultaneously evolved and the scientist finds plausible arguments for a certain thesis depending on his ideological background. In addition to that, finding an answer using methods of modern molecular genetics is unlikely because such a drastic genetic change within 10 to 20 years is not plausible. The attempt to explain the rise of psychiatric disorders as a result of an infection or electromagnetic waves has repeatedly failed.

A promising theory may be the "polyvagal theory" as proposed by SW Porges (Porges, 2009). It showed that our autonomous nervous system does not only control the heartbeat and peristalsis but also our social and emotional behavior. This mostly refers to the vagal efferents. Pediatric cardiologists are familiar with the Porges approach to measure the interaction between the brain and the heart by analyzing the HRV. The 24-hour ECG as an absolutely non-invasive method is an ideal way of researching this topic involving children.

Based upon the hypothesis that behavioural problems are accompanied by changes of the autonomic nervous system, we have performed analysis of HRV in 24 hours using Holter ECG's since the year 2005.

## 2.3. Comparison of Heart Rate Variability between Two Generations

On comparing the normal values of HRV in childhood from the years 1995-1997 as collected by Massin (Massin & von Bernuth, 1997) with our values from the years 2010 - 2012 (De Bock et al., 2013), it is remarkable that only the global HRV parameter SDNN lies within the normal distribution (Figure 2.2). In our control group it is however noticeable that the current rMSSD values lie in the lower part of normal distribution. Should this trend be confirmed by a larger study, then it has come, within the last decade, to a general decrease of vagal activity in childhood years. This loss of physiological, pre-pubertal vagal activity will - within the meaning of Porges polyvagal theory - have consequences on the social and emotional development of the children and correlation may not just be coincidental but possibly causal. According to Porges polyvagal theory this vagal shift may explain the increasing number of emotional disorders in children and probably also disorders in later life. Looking to the trend of vagal activity within lifetime as indicated in Figure 1.4 the decline of rMSSD starts from the maximum at puberty and ends at the end of life with the lowest values. The growing incidence of cardiovascular disease and depression in adults may be related to worsened vagal maturation in childhood when these diseases are characterized by low vagal activity.

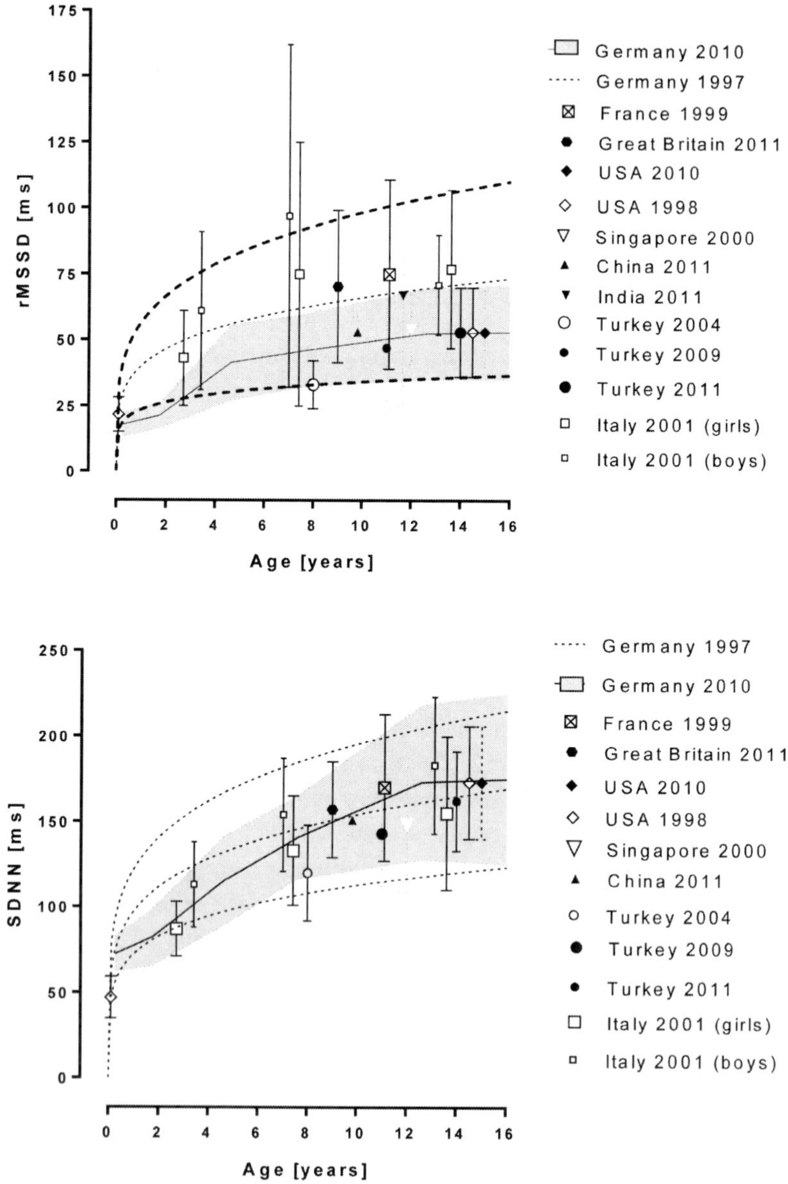


Figure 2.2. Comparison of HRV between two generations and different countries. The regression curves from Germany were published in 1997 and 2013.

## 2.4. International Comparison of HRV in Healthy Children

There are a large number of publications with HRV data from healthy children from all over the world. By collecting some of this data as illustrated in Figure 2.2 we found a reduced vagal activity indicated by the rMSSD values in children from United States in 1998 (Umetani et al., 1998) and 2010 (Zulfiqar et al., 2010a), from China in 2012 (Ma et al., 2011) and from Turkey published in 2004 (Unalacak et al., 2004), 2009 (Tascilar et al., 2009) and 2011(Akcaboy et al., 2011). The higher values as published from Germany in 1997 (Massin & von Bernuth, 1997) were measured in Great Britain in 2011 (Birch et al., 2012), France in 1999 (Butera et al., 1999) and India in 2011. The data from Italy published in 2001 (Silvetti et al., 2001) showed very high values in children with an age between four and twelve years. All these studies showed comparable heart rates and global heart rate variability indicated by SDNN. In summary the vagal shift in childhood started in the United States at least in 1998 and reaches Turkey, Singapore, China and Germany after the year 2000. Better HRV values were measured in children from Great Britain, France, Italy and India. Looking for the causes and consequences of this vagal shift, we analyzed HRV in children with new diseases in childhood and the effect of nutrition and sports.

## 2.5. HRV and Cardiovascular Risk

HRV analysis is routinely used for risk stratification in cardiology. Global heart rate variability (SDNN) and vagal activity (rMSSD) are reduced in patients with heart failure, hypertension and arrhythmias. Reduced HRV is proved as a strong predictor of arterial hypertension in the Framingham study (Jelinek et al., 2013) and in a large Indian cohort (Pal et al., 2012d). A shift of the autonomic nervous system to sympathetic dominance in childhood would explain the worldwide increase of blood pressure in childhood which cannot be explained by the increase of the body mass index alone (Wabitsch et al., 2002).

Recently we described a high incidence of ventricular tachycardia together with a reduced heart rate variability in a cohort of children with attention deficit disorder (Buchhorn & Christian, 2013a). Large observational studies about the risk of sudden cardiac death in children with ADHD could not find an increased risk of patients on methylphenidate but showed an increased baseline risk of patients without medication (Cooper et al., 2011a). As previously shown in adults with major depression these observations in children with ADHD may be evidence of an increased cardiovascular risk in patients with psychiatric disease due to autonomic imbalance (Stapelberg et al., 2012).

## 2.6. Road Map for Further Research

The attempt to explain fundamental changes in pediatric mental health with dysfunction of the autonomous nervous system is a bold hypothesis considering that practical consequences are currently still unknown. Nevertheless, the chosen methodological approach offers the unique opportunity to find an objective answer to the urgent questions concerning the cause of psychiatric and emotional disorders in children irrespective of ideological and educational concepts. Further studies examining the effects of several different interventions on the HRV should be referred to for this purpose. We have performed the following work up and plan further investigations as far as it is possible within the capacity of a small pediatric department with limited research funds:

1) Influence of nutrition, body mass index, caloric intake and especially the substitution with Omega 3 fatty acids on the HRV
2) Influence of physical activity and media usage on the HRV
3) Influence of growth and birth weight on the HRV (fetal programming)
4) Influence of pharmacological intervention on the HRV (Methylphenidate, beta-blockers, clonidine, growth hormone, caffeine etc)
5) Influence of educational interventions on the HRV
6) Influence of relaxation and biofeedback exercises on the HRV
7) Influence of different family constellations on the HRV
8) Further research on the evident regional differences in the incidence of pediatric psychiatric disorders by using the HRV (field studies)
9) Influence of specific psychotherapeutic interventions, e.g., the neuro-emotional integration through eye movement desensitization and reprocessing (EMDR) on the HRV, in particular in children with posttraumatic stress disorder

10) Influence of environmental toxins e.g., pollution, phthalates and intensity of information and communication technology usage on HRV

*Chapter 3*

# The Impact of Body Mass Index, Caloric Intake and Omega-3-Fatty Acids on HRV

## 3.1. Pathophysiology

I wish to show in this book that the "Big Three" of new morbidities in childhood - obesity, anorexia nervosa and attention deficit disorder – are each characterized by a specific pattern of autonomic imbalance. Looking for the cause of autonomic dysfunction in childhood, we realize that nutrition and micro nutrition have a high impact on HRV(Dippacher et al., 2014).

We performed a cross-sectional study comparing our HRV data from healthy children with a body mass index between >10$^{th}$ percentile and < 90$^{th}$ percentile and aged between 10 and 16 years, overweight children with a body mass index over 96$^{th}$ percentile, thin healthy children with a body mass index lower 10$^{th}$ percentile and children with a comparable body mass index due to anorexia nervosa. ANOVA analysis showed significant intergroup differences for heart rate ($p < 0.001$) and SDNN ($p < 0.001$). Post-hoc testing revealed that healthy thin children had normal heart rates and all in all normal HRV. As shown in Figure 3.1 children with anorexia nervosa had significantly lower heart rates ($p < 0.0001$) and obese children had significantly higher heart rates ($p = 0.033$). These differences came along with significantly higher global HRV expressed as SDNN in children with anorexia nervosa ($p < 0.0001$) and significantly lower SDNN in overweight children ($p = 0.002$). However, significantly decreased 24 hour SDNN values in overweight children were a consequence of smaller differences of heart rates between day and night values and this difference in overweight children was mainly derived from elevated heart rates at night. We found the strongest and highly significant relationship between SDNN and heart rate at night with r = 0.891 ($R^2 = 0.79$, $p < 0.001$). This data clearly indicate that global heart rate variability SDNN in children / adolescents is determined for the most part by heart rate during sleep.

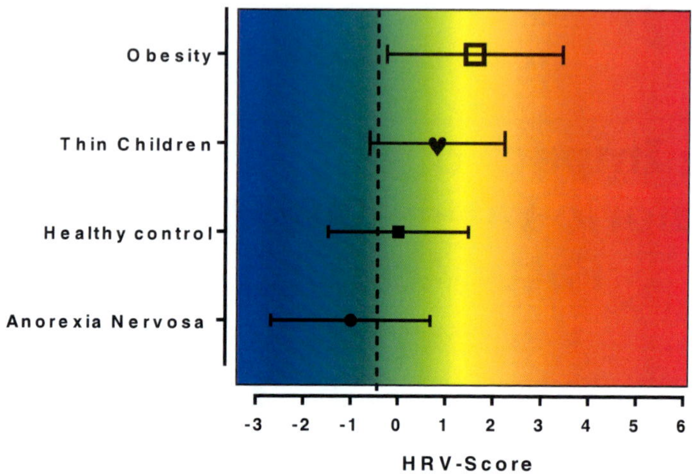


Figure 3.1. Autonomic balance indicated by our HRV-Score in children according to their nutritional state.

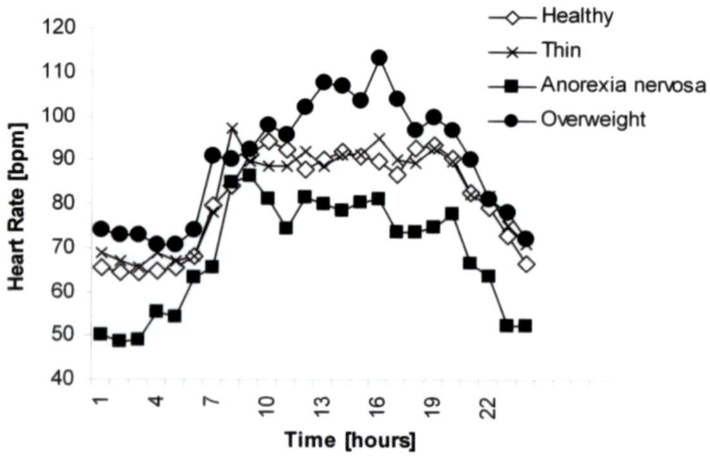


Figure 3.2. Circadian heart rate pattern in children according to their nutritional state.

## Table 3.1. HRV of children according to their nutritional state

| Table | Healthy Control | | Obesity | | | Thin Children | | | Anorexia Nervosa | | |
|---|---|---|---|---|---|---|---|---|---|---|---|
| | N= 52 | | N = 32 | | | N=16 | | | N=26 | | |
| Gender | 25♀ : 27♂ | | 15♀ : 17♂ | | | 10♀ : 6♂ | | | 22♀ : 4♂ | | |
| | Mean | +/- SD | Mean | +/- SD | p-value | Mean | +/- SD | p-value | Mean | +/- SD | p-value |
| Age | 12.8 | 1.7 | 12.3 | 2.1 | 0.17 | 12.9 | 1.9 | 0.68 | 15.0**** | 2.0 | <0.0001 |
| Height percentile [%] | 50.7 | 28.6 | 61.0 | 29.9 | 0.13 | 49.7 | 23.8 | 0.9 | 56.3 | 30.1 | 0.44 |
| Weight percentile [%] | 47.7 | 11.2 | 96.7*** | 6.2 | <0.0001 | 12.9 | 12.6 | <0.0001 | 20.6**** | 18.3 | <0.0001 |
| BMI percentile [%] | 45.9 | 23.7 | 98.5*** | 1.2 | <0.0001 | 3.8 | 3.3 | <0.0001 | 2.1**** | 4.7 | <0.0001 |
| Heart Rate Variability | | | | | | | | | | | |
| Heart rate [bpm] | 80.5 | 8.8 | 86.4 | 8.8 | 0.033 | 81.8 | 6.5 | 0.57 | 62.0**** | 11.3 | <0.0001 |
| SDNN [ms] | 182 | 47 | 145*** | 34 | 0.002 | 156 | 28 | 0.04 | 264**** | 65 | <0.0001 |
| rMSSD [ms] | 47 | 13 | 39** | 14 | 0.006 | 46 | 9 | 0.73 | 63**** | 18 | <0.0001 |
| TP 24h | 6625 | 3225 | 4400** | 2749 | 0.003 | 5843 | 2001 | 0.43 | 7868 | 3204 | 0.09 |
| VLF 24h | 3989 | 2662 | 2526** | 1905 | 0.008 | 3179 | 1390 | 025 | 4728 | 2456 | 0.24 |
| LF 24h | 1634 | 616 | 1103*** | 617 | 0.0002 | 1668 | 566 | 0.84 | 1794 | 650 | 0.3 |
| HF 24h | 835 | 331 | 694 | 388 | 0.079 | 908 | 290 | 0.44 | 1303**** | 467 | <0.0001 |
| HF/LF 24h | 0.53 | 0.17 | 0.65** | 0.23 | 0.006 | 0.57 | 0.16 | 0.39 | 0.77**** | 0.26 | <0.0001 |

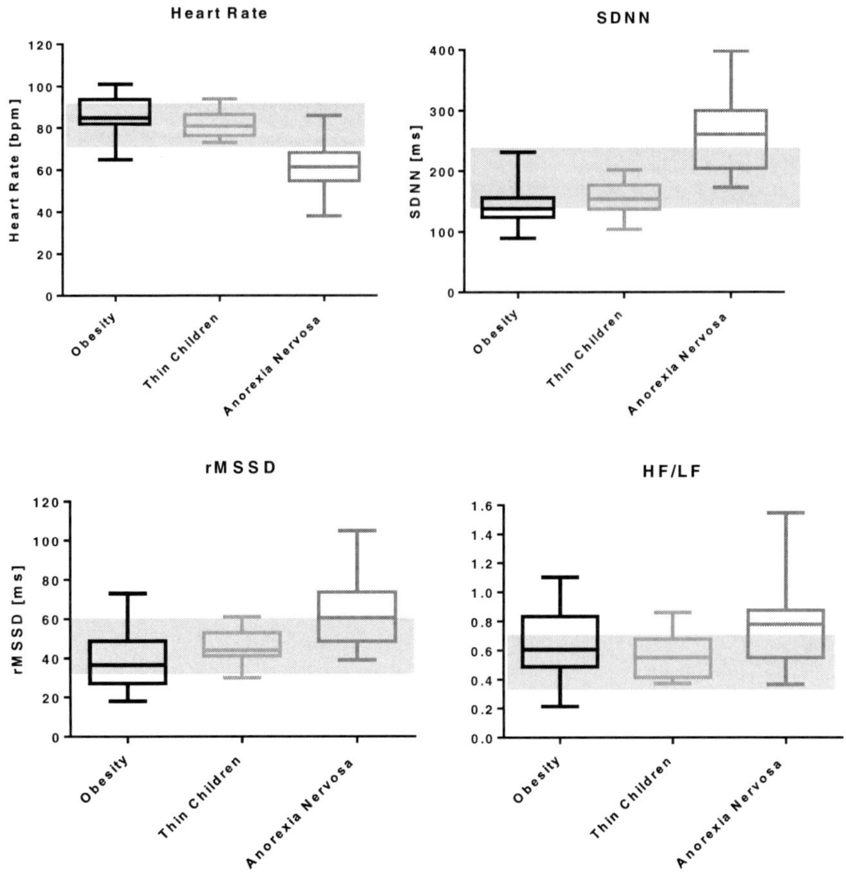


Figure 3.3. Autonomic balance of children according to their nutritional state indicated by the average heart rate, SDNN, rMSSD and HF to LF ratio of a 24 hour Holter ECG. The gray area indicates the mean ± one standard deviation of the healthy control group.

For a better understanding of the interaction between mean heart rate and HRV (Billman, 2013a) we have to realize that global HRV depends on heart rate showing a strong correlation during maturation of the autonomic nervous system from infancy to adulthood (Figure 3.4). This data lies on the same line in our group of healthy children published in 2013 and Massin's group of children published in 1997 despite a significant difference in rMSSD values. Within the same age group between 10 and 16 years all marks were lying again on one regression line but patients with anorexia nervosa, overweight and thin children were clustered (Figure 3.5.).

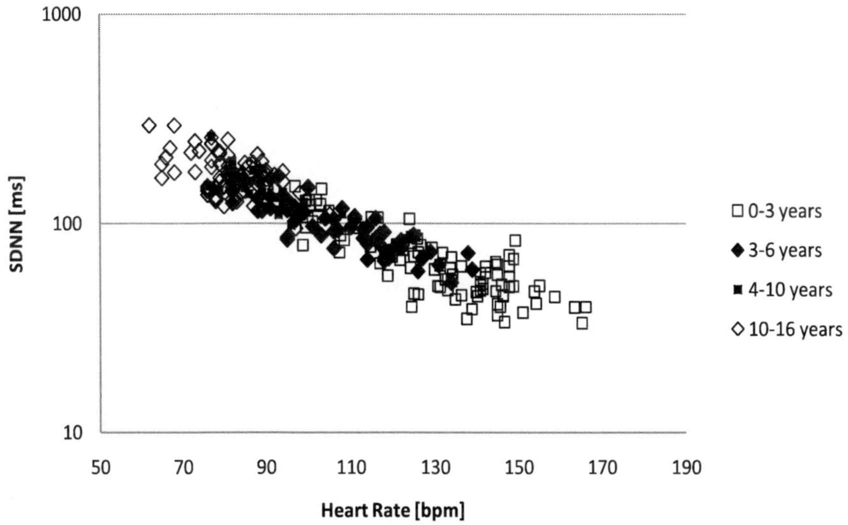


Figure 3.4. Mean heart rate and global HRV (SDNN) in 24 hour Holter ECG's of healthy children between birth and 16 years.

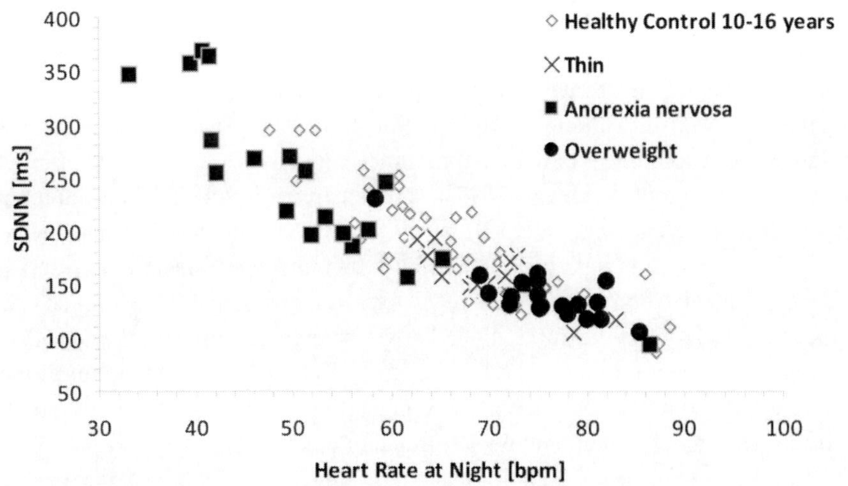


Figure 3.5. Mean heart rate at night and global HRV (SDNN) in 24 hour Holter ECG's of children between 10 and 16 years with respect to their nutritional state.

Based upon this strong relationship between heart rate and global HRV (SDNN) we are able to leave the "abstract world" of HRV analysis and the two dimensional thinking of the autonomic nervous system. Accumulating evidence clearly demonstrates that this assumption is naïve and greatly oversimplifies the complex non-linear interactions between the sympathetic and the parasympathetic divisions of the autonomic nervous system (Billman, 2013c). Most of these interpretations are based upon the short time HRV response to interventions that either increase or reduce autonomic neural activity in animal models. Our data now demonstrates the effect of specific interventions on long time HRV and circadian rhythm during the complex maturation of the autonomic nervous system in childhood.

Based upon this data, heart rate regulation in children not only results from changes in cardiac autonomic regulation but also from alterations of the intrinsic pacemaker rate. If one regards metabolic rate as the universal 'pacemaker' for biological processes (Glazier, 2014) then metabolism may drive the operating speed of closely related physiological functions (e.g. breathing and heart rhythm). G. Weitz et al. demonstrate that high resting energy expenditure is associated with lower long wave fluctuations (VLF) of heart rate in subjects with normal birth weight; the opposite can be seen in subjects with low birth weight (Weitz et al., 2013). Both the very low frequency component and the resting energy expenditure decline throughout life time. Further evidence indicates that metabolic rate does not necessarily drive food-intake rate, but conversely increased food intake may elevate metabolic rate. Thinking like an evolutionary biologist the correlation between caloric intake and heart rate during sleep seems to be part of the physiological regulation during hibernation. This relationship has been best studied in the regulation of food intake in mammalian hibernators reviewed by GL Florant et al. in 2011 (Florant & Healy, 2012): "... this form of self-induced anorexia hypothesized that annual fluctuations of food intake in these animals were likely the result of an endogenous 'sliding set-point' mechanism which sets a different 'ideal' body mass for each season, presumably regulated by hypothalamic control of food intake" (Mrosovsky & Powley, 1977). This regulation seems not to be related to the autonomic nervous system but to the hypothalamus-pituitary-adrenocortical connection (HPA axis) (Lo et al., 2008) and related suprachiasmatic nuclei as circadian clocks (Hastings et al., 2007).

Further we have to take into account three main sub-systems of the autonomic nervous system: the parasympathetic nervous system, sympathetic nervous system, and the "mysterious" enteric nervous system. Depending on the circumstances, these sub-systems may operate independently of each other or interact co-operatively. The enteric nervous system can operate autonomously and has the capacity to alter its response depending on such factors as bulk, nutrient composition and the microbiome.

*Taken together interpretation of HRV in children has to consider at least 4 qualities:*

1) The *intrinsic pacemaker rate* depends on age and caloric intake and is represented by heart rate, SDNN and Total Power (probably most of all by the very low frequency power). The intrinsic pacemaker rate predicts the baseline heart rate and seems to be related to the metabolic rate and is generated from the hypothalamus. The instantaneous heart rate regulation around this baseline heart rate depends on symapatho-vagal regulation.
2) The *circadian rhythm* generated by the suprachiasmatic nuclei and the hypothalamus-pituitary-adrenocortical connection (HPA axis).
3) The *parasympathetic activity* generated from specific nuclei in the central nervous system responsible for the "rest-and-digest" or "feed and breed" response that is represented by rMSSD, pNN50 and high frequency power. According to Porges polyvagal theory the "new vagus" is connected to the frontal cortex and represents social interaction as well as the so called executive functions (Diamond, 2012).
4) The *sympathetic activity* (e.g. generated by the limbic system) responsible to mobilize the "fight-or-flight" response. It is very difficult to estimate sympathetic activity with one HRV parameter like low frequency power or the HF to LF ratio. However we feel the quality "stress" if heart rate is high and HRV is low. The difficulty to define "stress" is one of the most methodological problematic issues in HRV analysis.

## 3.2. Obesity

Obesity in children today is an important forerunner of cardiovascular risk and is related to a dysfunction of the autonomic nervous system. This hypothesis was confirmed by several publications, recently in a prospective cross-sectional study (Baum et al., 2013). The pathophysiological pathway from autonomic imbalance and reduced HRV has been attributed to arterial hypertension (Thayer et al., 2010b;Pal et al., 2012c), heart failure (Buchhorn et al., 2002c) and sudden cardiac death (Vaseghi & Shivkumar, 2008).

As previously shown, obese children had elevated heart rates and lower SDNN values. The interpretation of these data is much more complicated because this effect cannot be explained by a simple autonomic shift to sympathetic dominance. Time domain analysis showed a parasympathetic withdrawal with lower rMSSD and pNN50. However these trends were not confirmed by the frequency domain analysis. In contrast LF values decreased, HF values were unchanged and the HF/LF ratio increased which has to be interpreted as a shift to parasympathic dominance. Taken together significant higher heart rates at night in overweight children cannot be explained by a simple autonomic shift in HRV analysis toward a sympathetic dominance. Obesity probably increases the intrinsic pacemaker rate indicated by higher heart rates and lower global HRV. The lower Total Power of the Fast Fourier Analysis is related in to a simultaneous decrease in VLF, LF and HF Power.

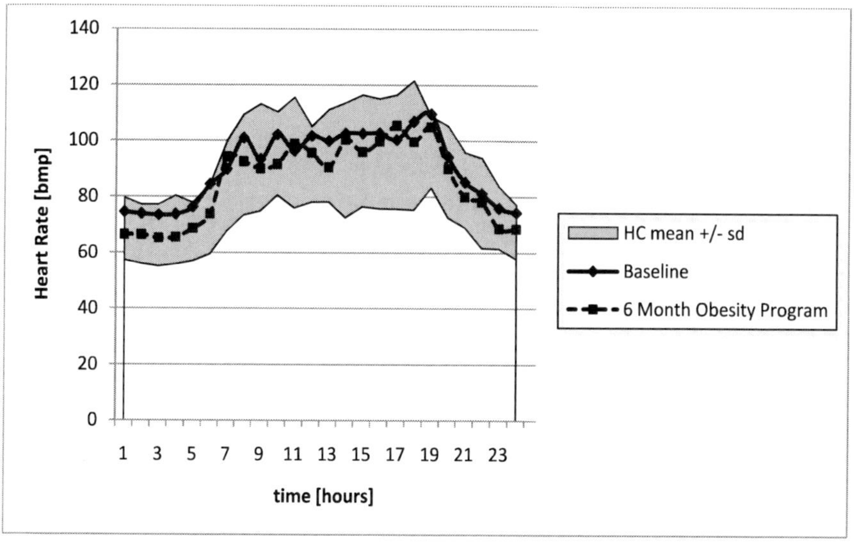


Figure 3.6. Circadian heart rate of 12 children who suffering from obesity with a BMI > 96% at baseline and after a 6 month childhood obesity program “KIDS”.

This model may explain the autonomic effects of an childhood obesity program “KIDS” in 12 children. After a 6 month high intensity education and physical training program we observed a significant decrease in heart rate and an increase in HRV indicated by SDNN and Total Power although the body mass index decreased only insignificantly. After a further six month low intensity training program the children’s HRV decreased again.

**Table 3.2. 24 hour HRV analysis of 12 children suffering from obesity with a BMI > 96% at baseline and after a 6 month childhood obesity program "KIDS"**

| | Baseline | | 6 Month Obesity Program | | |
|---|---|---|---|---|---|
| Parameters | N = 12 | | N = 12 | | |
| Gender | 3♀ : 9♂ | | 3♀ : 9♂ | | |
| | Mean | +/- SD | Mean | +/- SD | p-value |
| Age | 10,74 | 1,25 | 10,92 | 1,44 | 0,229 |
| Height percentile [%] | 77,08 | 18,06 | 80,25 | 15,88 | 0,175 |
| Weight percentile [%] | 98,25 | 2,60 | 96,42 | 3,18 | 0,014 |
| BMI percentile [%] | 98,75 | 1,66 | 96,42 | 4,52 | 0,099 |
| Heart rate [bpm] | 88,58 | 7,24 | 81,83 | 6,03** | 0,008 |
| Heart rate day [bpm] | 401,33 | 168,43 | 546,33 | 229,30 | 0,100 |
| Heart rate night [bpm] | 1061,67 | 497,20 | 1444,75 | 554,22* | 0,034 |
| SDNN [ms] | 150,08 | 33,63 | 170,58 | 40,92* | 0,033 |
| rMSSD [ms] | 39,67 | 9,83 | 47,17 | 9,46* | 0,013 |
| Total Power [$ms^2$] | 4281,25 | 1596,51 | 6368,75 | 2350,15** | 0,002 |
| High Frequency [$ms^2$] | 2350,08 | 923,81 | 3696,83 | 1790,02* | 0,013 |
| Low Frequencey [$ms^2$] | 1140,08 | 551,13 | 1640,08 | 635,55* | 0,016 |
| Very Low Frequency [$ms^2$] | 699,33 | 267,32 | 933,17 | 319,76** | 0,005 |
| HF/LF Ratio | 0,66 | 0,23 | 0,64 | 0,27 | 0,756 |

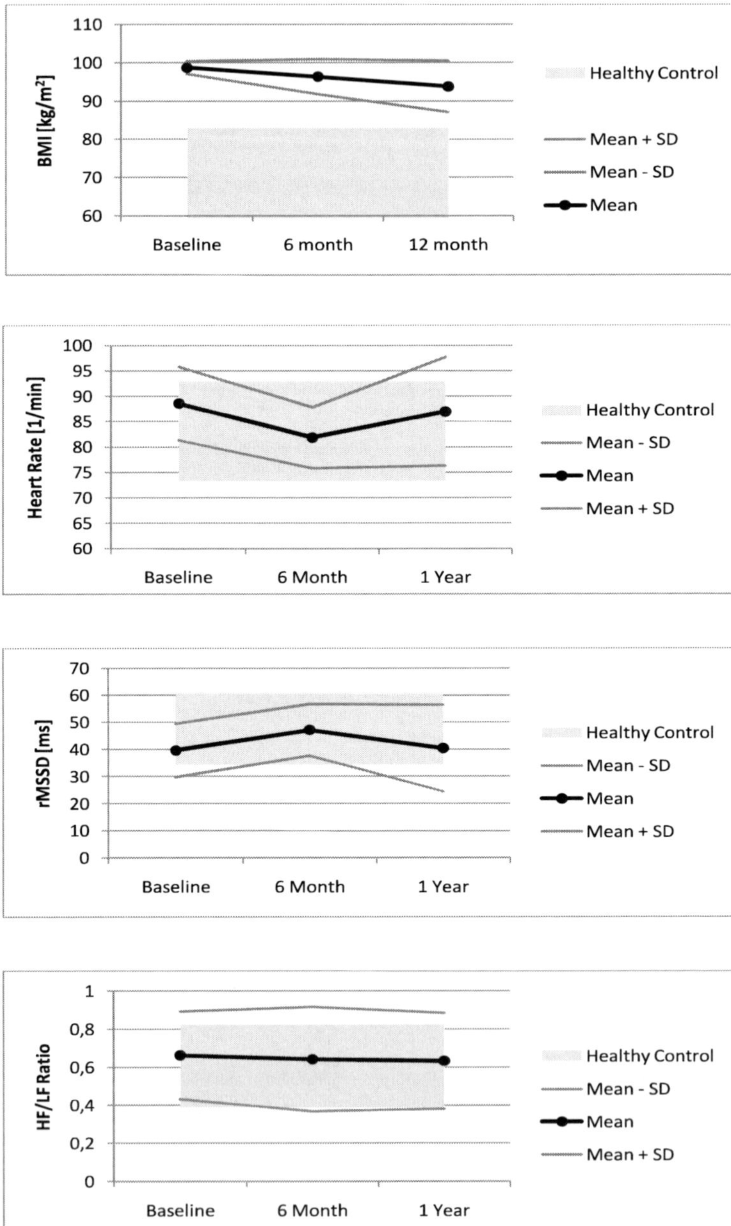


Figure 3.7. Effect of the childhood obesity program "KIDS" on BMI and 24 hour HRV. The significant HRV improvement after a 6 month intensive training was lost after further six months low intensity training - despitea lower BMI on average.

The Fast Fourier Analysis of 24 hour HRV show that the significant HRV improvement after 6 month intensive training was related to the increase of VLF Power with unchanged HF to LF ratio. This might be evidence increased caloric intake leads to an "hypermetabolic state" with higher heart rates at night and lower VLF power, and no clear effect on sympatho-vagal balance. If autonomic regulation worsened and VLF decreased again - despite the lower body mass indices – a majority of children of our KIDS program probably increase their caloric intake again during the low intensity training at the second half of the one year program.

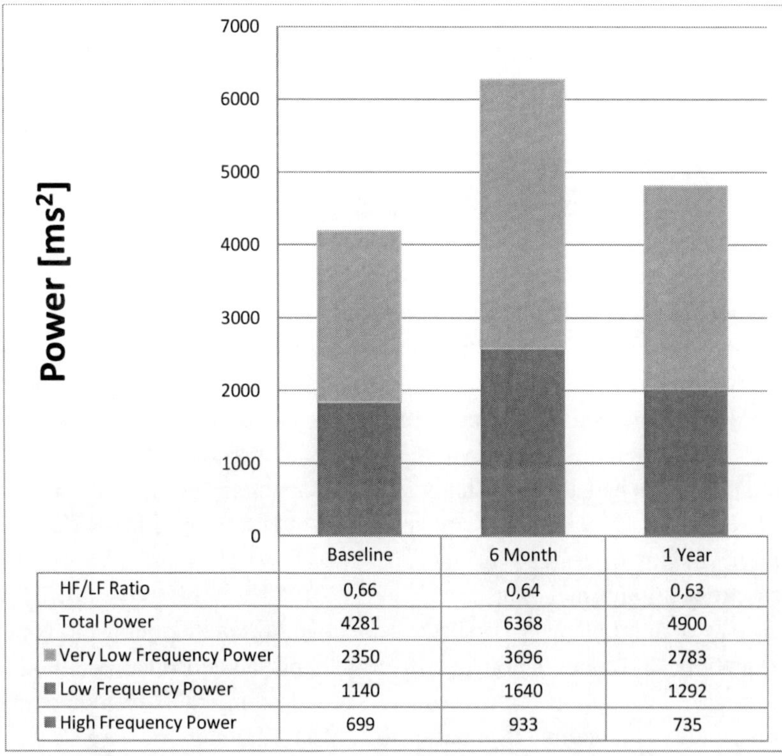


| | Baseline | 6 Month | 1 Year |
|---|---|---|---|
| HF/LF Ratio | 0,66 | 0,64 | 0,63 |
| Total Power | 4281 | 6368 | 4900 |
| Very Low Frequency Power | 2350 | 3696 | 2783 |
| Low Frequency Power | 1140 | 1640 | 1292 |
| High Frequency Power | 699 | 933 | 735 |

Figure 3.8. Effect of the childhood obesity program "KIDS" on Fast Fourier Analysis of 24 hour HRV. The significant HRV improvement after 6 month intensive training was related to the increase of VLF Power with unchanged HF to LF ratio.

Our data has further implication for cardiovascular risk stratification in obese children. As shown by Pal et al. (Pal et al., 2012a) a reduced HRV is a sign for pre-hypertension, and moreover, a reduced heart rate day to night ratio is a sign of vascular disease (Garcia-Ortiz et al., 2011) and a risk of all-cause mortality (Ben Dov et al., 2007). These insights open new therapeutic approaches to improve cardiovascular risk for example by a chrono-pharmacotherapy (Kaur et al., 2013) with a beta-blocker to decrease heart rate at night or to explain popular strategies like "sleeping well to stay slim" (Sokolovic et al., 2013). Moreover caloric reduction seems to be a very strong intervention to improve HRV and reduce cardiovascular risk (Weiss & Fontana, 2011). HRV analysis could clearly demonstrate to the patient the success of these interventions long before a BMI change.

Recently we realize that HRV is most of all reduced in obese children with metabolic syndrome indicated by hypertension and impaired glucose tolerance and lipid metabolism. Omega-3-fatty acids improve both - HRV and metabolic syndrome.

## 3.3. Anorexia Nervosa

Reviews today still show that there is no consistent view about the autonomic dysfunction in anorexia nervosa. Our data suggest that current BMI respectively nutritional state is not directly associated with HRV parameters. We agree at large with Petretta et al. (Petretta et al., 1997) who demonstrated normal HRV parameters in thin women compared to enhanced values in patients with anorexia nervosa. At hospital admission, all children with anorexia nervosa had the well-known parasympathetic dominance with low heart rate, high HRV parameters and a significant elevation of the HF/LF ratio. After one month of re-feeding and an average weight gain of 5 kg, HRV decrease to nearly normal values.

Girls with anorexia nervosa suffer from amenorrhea. In contrast to patients with functional normogonadotropic, hypothalamic amenorrhea, patients with amenorrhea due to anorexia nervosa showed a significant dysregulation in multiple HRV parameters (Bomba et al., 2014). The authors suggest that an anorexic biological spectrum including normogonadotropic-, hypogonado-tropic hypothalamic amenorrhea and anorexia nervosa might exist in adolescents, expressing itself on different levels of severity, including hormonal, autonomic and psychopathologiacal aspects with an origin in the hypothalamic regulation.

**Table 3.3. 24 hour HRV analysis of 16 children suffering from anorexia nervosa at hospital admission and one month re-feeding with an average weight gain of 5 kg**

| Parameter | Healthy control | | Anorexia Baseline | | | Anorexia Refeeding | | |
|---|---|---|---|---|---|---|---|---|
| | N= 37 | | N = 16 | | | N = 16 | | |
| Gender | 19♀ : 18♂ | | 13♀ : 3♂ | | | 13♀ : 3♂ | | |
| | Mean | +/- SD | Mean | +/- SD | p-value | Mean | +/- SD | p-value |
| Age | 14,0 | 1,1 | 14,8 | 2,2 | 0,139 | 14,9 | 2,2 | 0,112 |
| Height percentile [%] | 52,7 | 28,1 | 59,6 | 33,5 | 0,488 | 56,7 | 34,2 | 0,684 |
| Weight percentile [%] | 52,6 | 25,2 | 10,2 | 11,7 | <0.001 | 13,1 | 17,7 | <0.001 |
| BMI percentile [%] | 52,1 | 26,9 | 2,1 | 5,7 | <0.001 | 5,6 | 13,8 | <0.001 |
| Heart rate [bpm] | 82 | 9 | 62 | 9 | <0.001 | 74 | 10 | 0,022 |
| Heart rate day [bpm] | 113 | 39 | 66 | 21 | 0,004 | 91 | 37 | 0,318 |
| Heart rate night [bpm] | 53 | 17 | 31 | 7 | <0.001 | 37 | 13 | 0,053 |
| SDNN [ms] | 172 | 48 | 269 | 68 | <0.001 | 182 | 47 | 0,508 |
| RMSSD [ms] | 44 | 13 | 64 | 15 | <0.001 | 49 | 14 | 0,204 |
| Total Power [ms$^2$] | 5614 | 2919 | 7869 | 3012 | 0,018 | 5979 | 2836 | 0,68 |
| High Frequency [ms$^2$] | 758 | 327 | 1307 | 396 | <0.001 | 1009 | 501 | 0,09 |
| Low Frequencey [ms$^2$] | 1506 | 630 | 1747 | 605 | 0,199 | 1378 | 716 | 0,549 |
| Very Low Frequency [ms$^2$] | 3295 | 2124 | 4769 | 2332 | 0,039 | 3534 | 2176 | 0,72 |
| HF/LF Ratio | 0,5 | 0,14 | 0,8 | 0,27 | 0,001 | 0,81 | 0,42 | 0,015 |

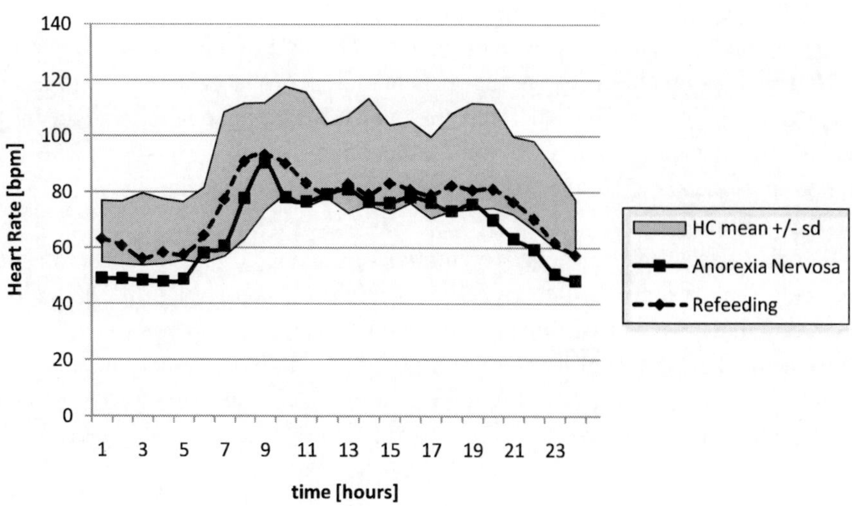


Figure 3.9. Circadian heart rate of 16 children suffering from anorexia nervosa at hospital admission and after one month re-feeding with an average weight gain of 5 kg.

At first view low heart rates and higher HRV and Total Power in children with anorexia nervosa may be explained by a simple autonomic shift in HRV analysis toward parasympathic dominance indicated by higher rMSSD, High Frequency Power and HF to LF ratio (Table 3.3). However during re-feeding we observed a quick "normalization" of HRV values but the HF to LF ratio remained elevated.

Again these autonomic effects during re-feeding may be explained by an increase of the intrinsic pacemaker rate with lower HRV indicated by lower SDNN and lower Total Power. In detail the decrease in Total Power is accompanied by lower HF, LF and VLF but with an unchanged HF to LF ratio (Fig. 3.10).

Our discovery of the rapid reaction of the autonomous nervous system to the increased caloric intake offers a possible explanation of hitherto contradicting results, most previous studies do not account for the caloric intake but just BMI. Given the rapid changes in HRV parameters some previous measurements may have detected the autonomic responses instead of the initial autonomic state of the illness. Moreover this rapid reaction shows that the autonomous nervous system is not a stable but a very dynamic system. Nonetheless HRV analysis and the known changes in anorexia nervosa is a helpful tool to differentiate in ambiguous cases of anorexia nervosa and habitual slimness.

These findings have important therapeutical implications for the treatment of anorexia nervosa. A consequent increase of caloric intake at the beginning of hospital stay by high caloric supplementation is probably necessary to reach the “autonomic switch” and interrupt the “hibernating circuit” induced by caloric restriction. In our view the “hibernating circuit” seems to delete the emotional memory of the patients, which is rewoken during nutritional rehabilitation.

This “flash back” of negative emotions may explain the resistance of the patients against nutrition therapy after reaching the caloric gain of 2000-2500 kcal/day after the first treatment week. Routine supplementation of omega-3-fatty acids, accompanied by sport and possibly beta-blockers in patients with extreme heart rate increases may help to smooth the “autonomic switch” and help the patient to tolerate the loss of the “vagal brake”.

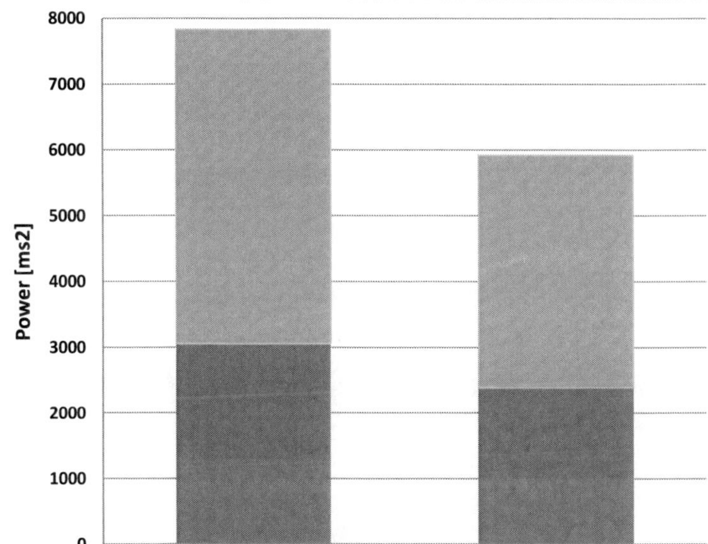


| | Anorexia Nervosa | Refeeding |
|---|---|---|
| HF/LF | 0,80 | 0,81 |
| VLF | 4769 | 3534 |
| LF | 1747 | 1377 |
| HF | 1307 | 1009 |

Figure 3.10. 24 hour Fast Fourier Analysis of 16 children suffering from anorexia nervosa at hospital admission and after one month re-feeding with an average weight gain of 5 kg.

Figure 3.11 shows a case study of a 16 year old girl with diagnosed anorexia nervosa with extreme low body weight (26.1 kg, BMI 10.3 kg/m², -8.4 SDS) before and while re-feeding according to the NICE protocol. It was the second hospitalization of this girl for anorexia nervosa but this time the illness was worse than the first time. After one week of re-feeding body weight rose just one kilogram (27.1 vs. 26.1 kg, BMI 10.9 vs. 10.5 kg/m²) but HRV parameters responded more and immediately: the mean heart rate rose about 13 bpm (71 vs. 53 bpm), while SDNN was divided in half (157 vs. 330 ms). rMSSD declined simultaneously (49 vs. 66 ms). In frequency domain analysis VLF (2589 vs. 4087), LF (824 vs. 990), HF (1018 vs. 1052) and HF/LF-ratio (1.24 vs. 1.54) declined too. After two weeks of re-feeding the change in weight outreached the new changes in HRV parameters (+1.4 kg, BMI 12.3 kg/m², heart rate 73 bpm, SDNN 130 ms, rMSSD 48 ms). After 7.5 weeks of treatment the girl weighted 37.1 kg (+ 11 kg, BMI 14.95 kg/m²).

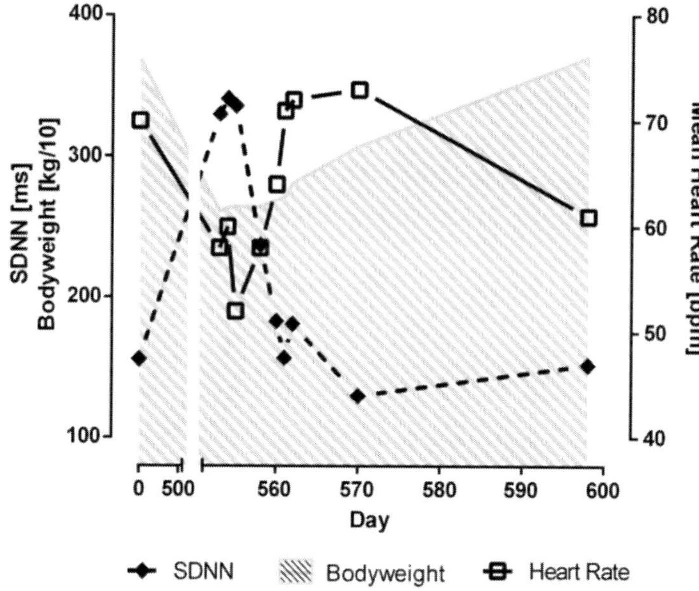


Figure 3.11. Case study of a 16 year old girl with anorexia nervosa and extreme low body weight (26.1 kg, BMI 10.3 kg/m², -8.4 SDS) before and during re-feeding according to the NICE protocol.

After this case we changed our therapeutic protocol with caloric and vitamin B supplementation according to the NICE protocol (Judges et al., 2012). We try to weaken the autonomic switch to sympathetic dominance with omega 3 fatty acid supplementation (Ayton et al., 2004) and biofeedback training (Scolnick et al., 2014). We observed an improved weight gain in additional 16 children after this change of protocol compared to our own historical data (Figure 3.12). We also compared our retrospective data with published interventional studies (Rocks et al., 2014): Age (14.8±1.8 years) and body mass index (14.1±1.6 kg/m$^2$) were comparable to these studies. Weight gain was the best with exclusively orally fed patients (Figure 3.13). Weight gain was comparable to the patients with additional nasogastric tube feeding (NGS) and better than the patients with additional parenteral nutrition (PN). In contrast to these interventions none of our patients need antianxiety medications.

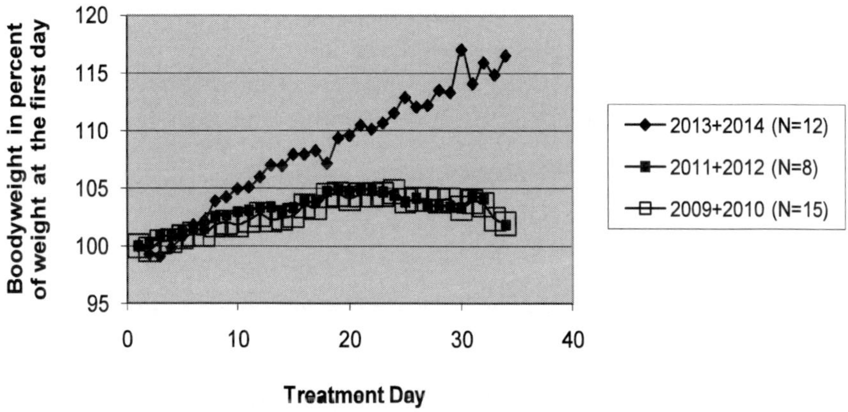


Figure 3.12. Weight gain of children with anorexia nervosa during the first month of hospital stay. There is a significant improvement of weight gain after changing the re-feeding protocol (NICE) in 2013 and 2014.

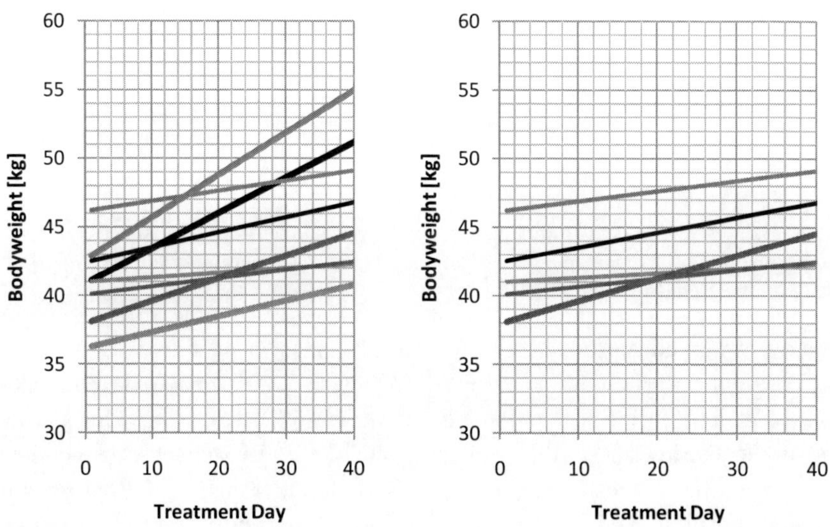


Figure 3.13. Comparison of weight gain in 4 retrospective, intervention studies during initiation of re-feeding in underweight children and adolescent with anorexia nervosa. Our results (red) after introduction of the modified NICE protocol show the best weight gain in exclusively orally fed patients (right diagram). Our results are comparable to additional nocturnal nasogastric feeding (green and black) and better than additional parenteral nutrition (blue) despite the lowest mean body mass index at the time of therapy initiation (14.1±1.6 kg/m$^2$) (left diagram).

However four patients had an early relapse of the starvation syndrome and needed a further hospital stay after 80 days on average. Although the mean loss of bodyweight is only 1.3 kg the average autonomic regulation was at the same as at the first admission with bradycardia and high rMSSD values (Figure 3.13).

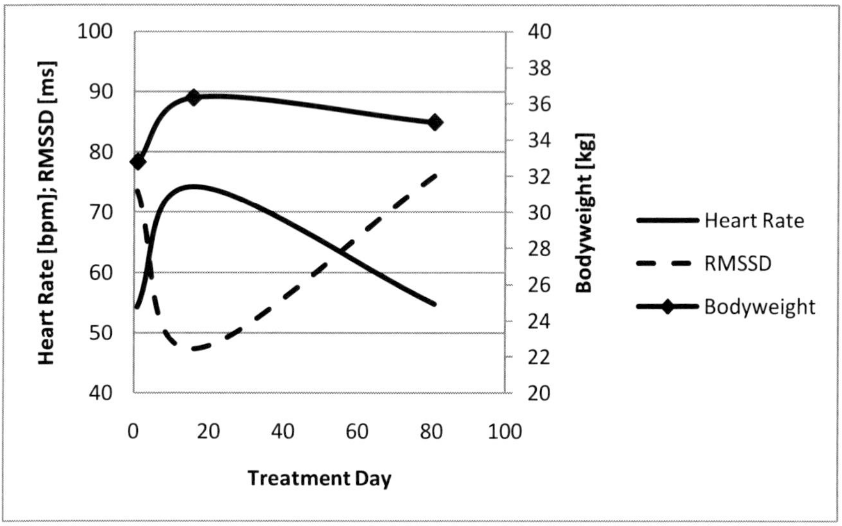


Figure 3.14. Average data from 4 patients with anorexia nervosa after successful re-feeding from 32.8 to 36.3 kg at day 16 and a relapse of starvation at day 80 with a mean bodyweight of 35 kg.

We observed reproducible autonomic changes in patients with Anorexia Nervosa during follow up as indicated in Figure 3.15. Compared to a healthy control patient during the initial state of starvation, HRV is very high at day and night. During successful re-feeding the same girl showed a sympathetic shift to normal values at day. Another girl during longtime follow up with multiple hospital stays showed a loss of vagal acitivty at day with extreme high HRV at night (albeit overestimated by technical aliasing). This “autonomic scare” has been described by M. Lachish et al. (Lachish et al., 2009), but I am not sure if this sympathetic regulation is not the cause of the disease prior to starvation. In the sense of a learning model the children had learned to treat their emotional stress by starvation. I am deeply convinced that Anorexia Nervosa is preventable by the consequent treatment of emotional stress and autonomic dysfunction in children for example after traumas (sexual abuse, familial conflicts) or a genuine stress diseases like attention deficit disorder.

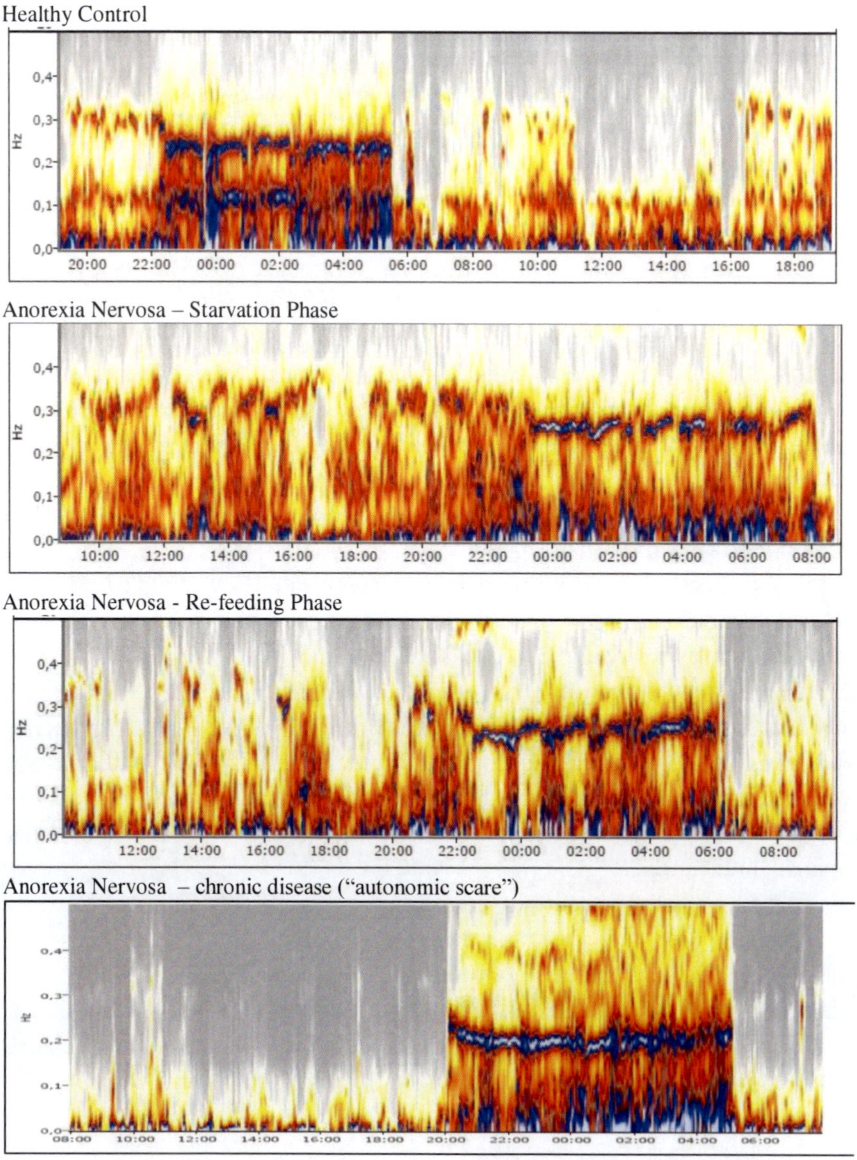


Figure 3.15. "Fire of Life" ™ pictures of children with anorexia nervosa in the starvation phase, during re-feeding and longtime follow up compared to a healthy control.

## 3.4. Omega 3 Fatty Acids

Omega 3 fatty acids consistently produce statistically significant reductions in baseline heart rate that are accompanied by increase in HRV (McLennan, 2014). Recent data strongly suggest that intrinsic changes in pacemaker rate may play a more important role in omega 3 fatty acid induced heart rate reductions than do changes in cardiac autonomic regulation.

There is an increasing evidence that supplementation of omega 3 fatty acids have beneficial effects in children with cognitive disorders like ADHD (Widenhorn-Muller et al., 2014). Further evidence also exists about the beneficial effects in adults with arrhythmias (Billman, 2012;Billman, 2013b). We observed severe autonomic dysfunction in children with somatoform disorders such as "fatigue syndrome" (Boneva et al., 2007) and fibromyalgia (Staud, 2008) with little pharmacological options. With respect to the therapeutic effects of omega 3 fatty acids in prospective trials and the well-known effects on HRV we used omega 3 fatty acid supplementation in 19 children with these disorders and monitored 24 hour HRV prior to supplementation and again, on average, three month later. We used different preparations with 1-2g fish oil per day. As shown in the table, there were highly significant effects on heart rate at night and HRV. If most of these children had elevated heart rate at night we interpret a normalization of heart rates at night as a beneficial effect, however most of all, in children with arrhythmias we observed impressive clinical benefits. The effect of omega 3 fatty acids on circadian heart rates is illustrated in Figure 3.15. Particularly when given in the morning prior to breakfast there is an impressive decrease of heart rates between midnight and early morning that is more pronounced compared to pharmacological therapies with beta- blockers and other antiarrhythmic drugs.

Taken together omega 3 fatty acids seem to have highly significant effects on intrinsic pacemaker rate and HRV in children with arrhythmias and somatoform disorders that may be related to their beneficial clinical effects. A Fast Fourier Analysis demonstrating higher total power and significant elevations of all frequencies with little effects on sympatho-vagal balance measured by the LF/HF ratio, indicates that omega 3 fatty acids improve the intrinsic pacemaker rate (Figure 3.16).

**Table 3.4. 24 hour HRV analysis of 19 children suffering from arrhythmias, attention deficit disorder or chronic fatigue syndrome at baseline and after 3 month omega 3 fatty acid supplementation**

| | Baseline | | Omega 3 fatty acid | | |
|---|---|---|---|---|---|
| | N= 19 | | | | |
| Gender | 10♀ : 9♂ | | | | |
| | Mean | +/- SD | Mean | +/- SD | p-value |
| Age | 13 | 4 | | | |
| Heart rate [bpm] | 96 | 11 | 85**** | 10 | <0.0001 |
| Heart rate day [bpm] | 102 | 13 | 95* | 12 | 0.0269 |
| Heart rate night [bpm] | 85 | 16 | 71**** | 9 | <0.0001 |
| SDNN [ms] | 127 | 49 | 148** | 32 | 0.0023 |
| rMSSD [ms] | 27 | 16 | 38*** | 11 | 0.0005 |
| TP 24h | 3201 | 2246 | 4608*** | 1883 | 0.0009 |
| VLF 24h | 1926 | 1462 | 2634** | 1410 | 0.0073 |
| LF 24h | 836 | 614 | 1224** | 577 | 0.0028 |
| HF 24h | 396 | 288 | 688**** | 312 | <0.0001 |
| HF/LF 24h | 0.5 | 0.26 | 0.61* | 0.26 | 0.0037 |

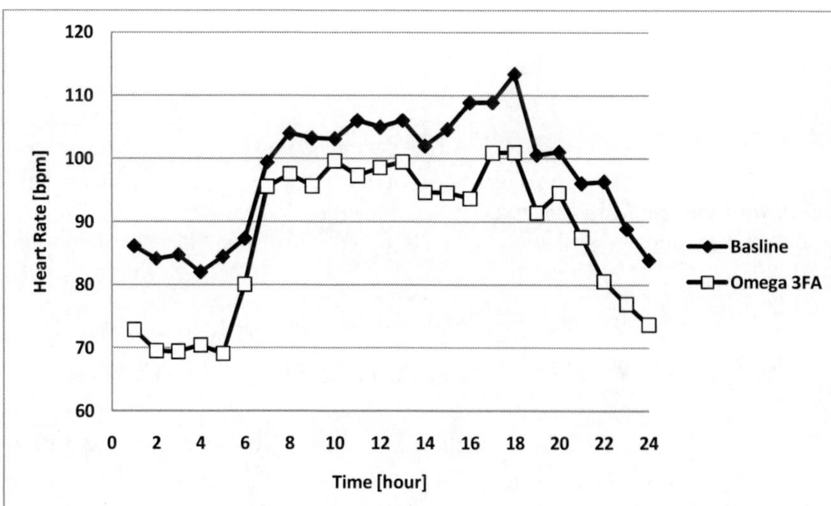


Figure 3.16. 24 hour circadian heart rate of 19 suffering from arrhythmias, attention deficit disorder or chronic fatigue syndrome at baseline and after 3 month omega 3 fatty acid supplementation

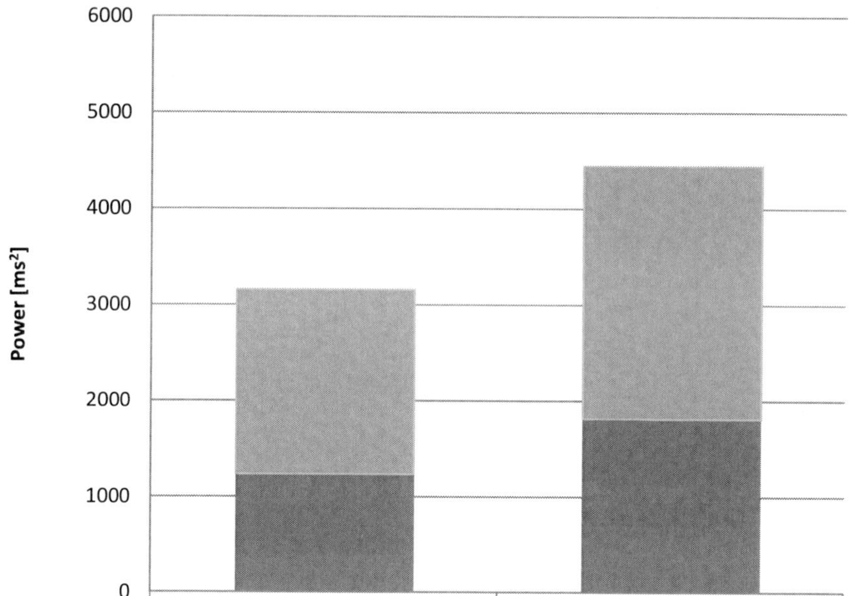


| | Baseline | Omega-3-FA |
|---|---|---|
| HF/LF | 0,50 | 0,61 |
| Total Power | 3201 | 4608 |
| VLF | 1926 | 2634 |
| LF | 836 | 1124 |
| HF | 396 | 688 |

Figure 3.17. Fast Fourier Analysis of omega-3-fatty acid supplementation effect of 19 children with autonomic dysfunction. The significant HRV improvement after 3 month was related to the increase of VLF, LF and HF Power with a slight increase of the HF to LF ratio.

## 3.5. HRV and Environmental Toxins

The interplay between fish consumption and mercury exposure most of all in pregnant women is complicated. Mercury exposure during childhood seems to affect HRV among Nunavik Inuit children of school age (Valera et al., 2012). However the FDA's new advice conclude that pregnant and nursing women should be advised to eat fish to benefit from naturally occurring omega 3 fatty acids, to avoid fish with high levels of mercury and other contaminants, and, if possible, to choose fish with high levels of omega 3 fatty acids

(Wenstrom, 2014). However other environmental toxins seem to be more important than mercury from sea food:

**Bisphenol A** (BPA) is a high-volume production chemical with in impact on HRV. Urinary BPA concentration reduces rMSSD and is related to hypertension (Bae et al., 2012).

Several studies report on the association between short term exposure to ambient air pollution and HRV. An increase in particulate matter with aerodynamic diameter of 10 µm or less (**$PM_{10}$**) or 2.5 µm or less (**$PM_{2.5}$**) is associated with a significant reductions in time-domain and in frequency-domain measurements (SDNN and rMSSD) (Pieters et al., 2012). The Multi-Ethnic Study of Atherosclerosis showed that autonomic dysfunction may be a mechanism through which **particulate air pollution** affects cardiovascular risk, especially among persons with metabolic syndrome (Park et al., 2010). Occupational exposure to environmental **tobacco smoke** may decrease heart rate variability (Zhang et al., 2013).

In contrast short-time exposure to electromagnetic fields emitted by mobile phones does not affect cardiac autonomic modulation in healthy subjects (Barutcu et al., 2011). There seems to be no immediate negative effect of media consumption on HRV in childhood (see Figure 5.1, 5.2 and 5.3). However there is growing evidence **that intensity of information and communication technology (ICT)** usage in childhood have an effect on quality of sleep and HRV (Lin et al., 2014;Ononogbu et al., 2014). Means, adjusted for gender, age and BMI of SDNN (99.05 versus 114.12 ms, p=0.002) and rMSSD (69.87 versus 82.61ms, p=0.008) are significantly lower in high ICT users compared to low ICT users (N=61).

Taken together particulate air pollution and intensity information and communication technology usage seems to be the most important environmental “toxin” to reduce HRV in childhood. Omega-3 fatty acid supplements offer protection against the adverse cardiac and lipid effects associated with air pollution exposure (Tong et al., 2012).

*Chapter 4*

# HRV and Mental Health

## 4.1. HRV in Children with ADHD and Learning Difficulties

Children receiving methylphenidate (MPH) for AD(H)D are seen by pediatric cardiologists on a routine basis due to the potential risk of cardiac arrhythmias. Since 2005, we have added 24 hour ECG to the routine diagnostics consisting of ECG, measurement of blood pressure and echocardiography. The systematic analysis of the HRV of 12 patients before methylphenidate therapy and 19 patients of the same age group under methylphenidate treatment revealed in 2010 surprisingly unequivocal results (Buchhorn et al., 2012a): Compared to healthy control patients, children with AD(H)D with or without methylphenidate treatment have a higher mean heart rate, lower sNN50 values likewise the rMSSD values indicated lower vagal activity (Table 4.1). The circadian analysis of the HRV showed an extensive reduction of circadian vagal activity measured as sNN50 in children with AD(H)D prior to methylphenidate therapy most of all at night (Figure 4.1). These data are in good accordance with a huge number of publications about ADHD and sleep disturbances. More over low sleep quality has an impact on HRV (Michels et al., 2013) and may be improved by omega-3-fatty acid supplementation (Montgomery et al., 2014). In addition, we observed a highly significant reduction of elevated heart rates at night in children who received omega-3-fatty acid supplementation for arrhythmias or somatoform disorders (chapter 3.4). Recent randomized trials showed a beneficial clinical effect of omega-3-fatty acid supplementation in children with AD(H)D and learning difficulties.

These results, if confirmed by prospective studies, are of major clinical and pathophysiological significance. They show that the HRV analysis in 24-hour ECG can be used as an objective bio marker for AD(H)D. Moreover, it may serve to monitor methylphenidate therapy (see chapter 8.4.).

**Table 4.1. HRV Data from children with AD(H)D before and after treating with methylphenidate (MPH)**

| | Healthy Control | ADHD - MPH | ADHD + MPH |
|---|---|---|---|
| N | 19 | 12 | 19 |
| Age [years] | 10.8 ± 3.5 | 10.8 ± 2.0 | 10.6 ± 2.8 |
| Height [cm] | 145 ± 19 | 143 ± 15 | 141 ± 15 |
| Bodyweight [kg] | 40 ± 14 | 35 ± 10 | 34 ± 10 |
| BMI [kg/m2] | 18 ± 3 | 17 ± 2 | 17 ± 2 |
| Mean Heart Rate [bpm] | 85 ± 10 | 94 ± 9** | 90 ± 8* |
| Minimal Heart Rate [bpm] | 58 ± 7 | 64 ± 9* | 58 ± 5 |
| Maximal Heart Rate [bpm] | 158 ± 25 | 177 ± 16* | 171 ± 17* |
| pNN50 [%] (vagal activity) | 21.5 ± 9.0 | 6.5 ± 2.7*** | 14.2 ± 6.9** |
| rMSSD [ms] (vagal activity) | 44 ± 10 | 26 ± 4*** | 37 ± 8** |
| SDNN [ms] (global HRV) | 146 ± 30 | 136 ± 41 | 151 ± 24 |

Data are shown as mean ± standard deviation.
*P-Value < 0.05; ** P- Value < 0.01; ***P- Value < 0.001.

To investigate HRV in children with respect to their school success we compare the 24 hour HRV data from 14 random students of the local high school with the data of 13 random children of a local school for children with learning difficulties. As shown in Tab. 4.2 age is comparable but the body mass index is higher in children with learning difficulties due to the higher incidence of obesity in this group. There is a significantly higher HRV in high school students within the normal range and significantly reduced values for SDNN and vagal activity indicated by rMSSD and pNN50 in children with learning difficulties. This data for children with learning difficulties may include untreated children with AD(H)D and it may be that some of their learning difficulties are related to untreated AD(H)D.

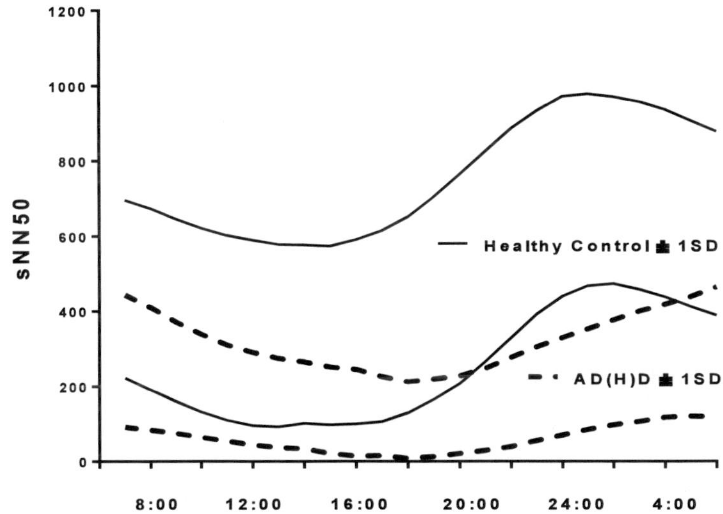


Figure 4.1. Circadian rhythm of vagal activity indicated by the parameter sNN50 in healthy children and in children with AD(H)D prior to medical therapy.

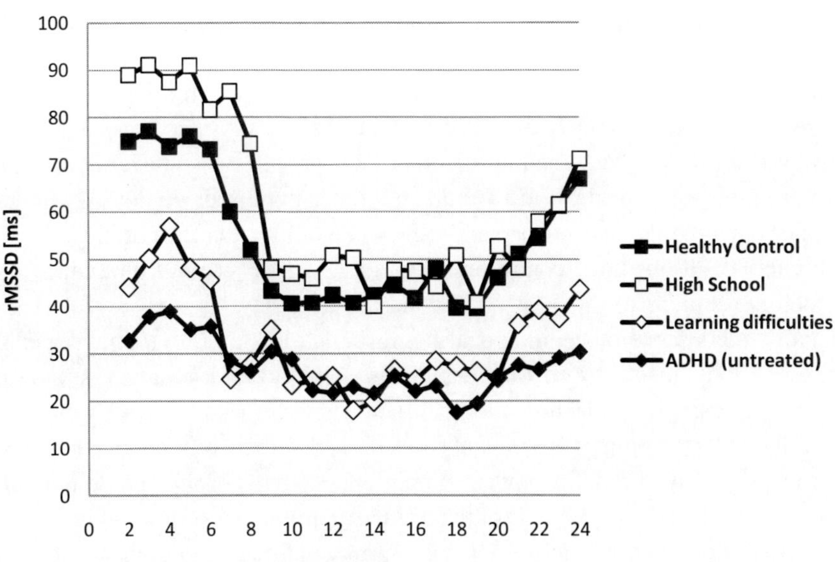


Figure 4.2. 24 hour vagal activity (rMSSD) from 14 unselected students of the local high school with the data of 13 unselected children of a local school for children with learning difficulties. The data of a healthy control group and children with untreated ADHD are included.

**Table 4.2. HRV data from children according to their school success**

| | Healthy Control | High School | Learning Difficulties |
|---|---|---|---|
| N | 71 | 14 | 13 |
| Age [Years] | 12.8 ± 1.7 | 12.6 ± 1.6 | 13.0 ± 1.5 |
| BMI [kg/qm] | 18.5 ± 2.5 | 18.9 ± 3.4 | 25.9 ± 6.1** |
| Mean Heart Rate [bpm] | 81 ± 8 | 83 ± 7 | 89 ± 6* |
| pNN50 [%] | 26.4 ± 11.0 | 25.2 ± 8.9 | 14.5 ± 9.1** |
| rMSSD [ms] | 46.9 ± 12.5 | 44 ± 9 | 33 ± 10** |
| SDNN [ms] | 173.7 ± 44.7 | 199 ± 44 | 139 ± 22*** |

Data is shown as Mean ± SD. Statistical *$P < 0.05$; ** $P < 0.001$; ***$P < 0.0001$.

## 4.2. HRV in Children with Somatoform Disorders

"A somatic symptom disorder, formerly known as a somatoform disorder, is a mental disorder characterized by physical symptoms that suggest physical illness or injury – symptoms that cannot be explained fully by a general medical condition or by the direct effect of a substance, and are not attributable to another mental disorder. In people who have a somatic symptom disorder, medical test results are either normal or do not explain the person's symptoms, and history and physical examination do not indicate the presence of a medical condition that could cause them. Symptoms are sometimes similar to those of other illnesses and may last for several years. Usually, the symptoms begin appearing during childhood (http://en.wikipedia.org/wiki/Somatic_symptom_disorder). In childhood somatic symptom disorder occurs as stomach or thoracic pain – and/or headache. Also multiple pains which is - sometimes misinterpreted as rheumatism - characterized as fibromyalgia syndrome. Another important patient group predominantly adolescents, is patients with chronic fatigue syndrome, sometimes after a virus infection like infectious mononucleosis. In most affected children we observe a significant autonomic dysfunction indicated by low HRV in 24 hour Holter ECG's (table 4.3.). Like shown in adults with chronic fatigue (Boneva et al., 2007) and fibromyalgia (Staud, 2008) these children have elevated heart rates, particularly at night. These finding explain our therapeutical approach to lower heart rate with beta-blockers and/or omega 3 fatty acids. To treat a child with a severe somatoform disorder is like "driving in a dust storm" but when this very difficult therapy is successful we can always measure a significant decrease of average heart rate at night. HRV analysis helps us to get a proper diagnosis and prove a sometimes unusual therapy. However, up to this point of research, we have not identified a specific autonomic dysfunction in children with chronic abdominal pain.

**Table 4.3. 24 hour HRV analyses of 14 children with severe somatoform disorders: chronic fatigue syndrome (N=12) or fibromyalgia (N=2)**

| | Healthy Control | | Somatoform Disorder | | |
|---|---|---|---|---|---|
| | N= 52 | | N = 14 | | |
| Gender | 25♀ : 27♂ | | 8♀ : 6♂ | | p-value |
| | Mean | +/- SD | Mean | +/- SD | |
| Age | 12.8 | 1.7 | 14.1* | 2.5 | 0.03 |
| Heart rate [bpm] | 80.5 | 8.8 | 98.0**** | 2.8 | < 0.0001 |
| SDNN [ms] | 182 | 47 | 96**** | 8 | < 0.0001 |
| rMSSD [ms] | 47 | 13 | 22**** | 3 | < 0.0001 |
| TP 24h | 6625 | 3225 | 2111**** | 481 | < 0.0001 |
| VLF 24h | 3989 | 2662 | 1197**** | 275 | < 0.0001 |
| LF 24h | 1634 | 616 | 626**** | 116 | 0.0005 |
| HF 24h | 835 | 331 | 298**** | 86 | < 0.0001 |
| HF/LF 24h | 0.53 | 0.17 | 0.81** | 0.37 | 0.136 |

## 4.3. HRV and Neurodevelopment

Evidence suggests that reduced HRV time domain parameters close to birth are associated with cerebral palsy diagnosis at the age of three years (Amichai & Katz-Leurer, 2014). It is unclear if autonomic dysfunction in infancy per se impairs neurodevelopment as shown in infants with heart failure due to congenital heart defects (Ravishankar et al., 2013). A lower vagal activity in patients with epilepsy is related to the failure of anticonvulsants and sudden unexpected death in epilepsy (see chapter 10)(Lotufo et al., 2012). Protection of the autonomic nervous system in early infancy will be a new promising therapeutic target to improve neurodevelopmental outcome in children with severe disease like congenital heart disease, prematurity and malnutrition.

*Chapter 5*

# Sports and HRV

Initially, we are highly motivated to improve HRV in children through sports (Henje et al., 2009) but have been disappointed with the inconsistent benefits. Accordingly a recently published metaanalysis from randomized controlled trials does not support the hypothesis that physical training improves HRV in healthy children (da Silva et al., 2014). However other groups showed benefits of sport on HRV in children e.g. Diabetes mellitus (Jaiswal et al., 2013), obesity (Gutin et al., 2005) or Down syndrome (Giagkoudaki et al., 2010). For these groups, it is probable that exercise has a positive effect on cardiac autonomic system in children who initially had a low HRV.

For a better understanding of the immediate effects of sports on HRV in children we compared the 24 hour HRV in 14 healthy children in one day with high intensity sports to another day with intensive media consumption. The heart rates (Figure 5.1) showed the expected effect of physical activity between 14:00 and 16:00 but compared to media usage slightly higher heart rates in the following night. This effect was caused by lower vagal activity indicated by pNN50 and rMSSD values. If we compare the seven children with the highest HRV with the seven children with the lowest HRV, vagal suppression indicated by the rMSSD value after sports persists until the next morning in the children with the low baseline HRV (Figure 5.2). The children with high HRV reach their rMSSD baseline just 4 hours after the same athletic exertion (Figure 5.3). These data clearly indicate a shorter stress recovery time in children with high HRV compared to those with low HRV. Our data are in good accordance with the hypothesis of Weber et al., that low vagal tone was associated with impaired recovery of cardiovascular, endocrine, and immune markers in healthy probands. The group posits reduced resting HRV as a risk marker for future cardiovascular and other stress-related disease (Weber et al., 2010).

Change for consistent legend

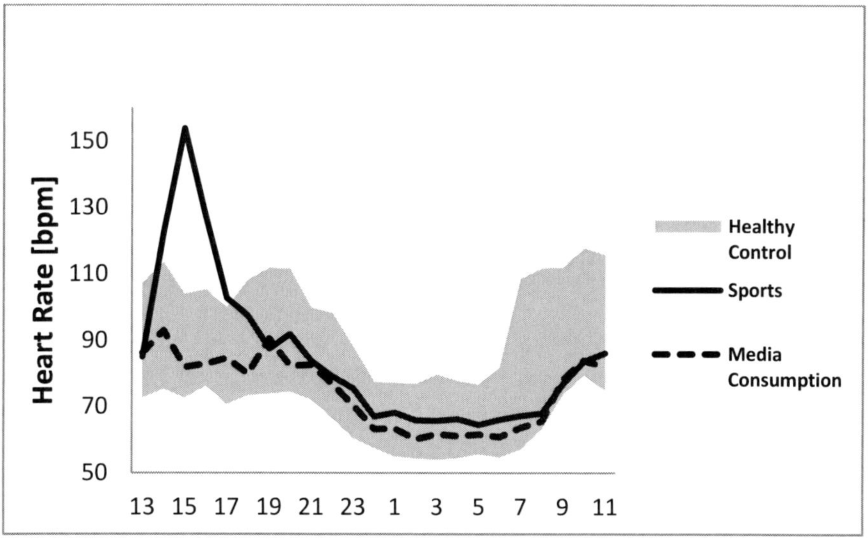


Figure 5.1. The effect of physical activity between 14:00 and 16:00 (compared to media consumption) on heart rate in 14 healthy high school children.

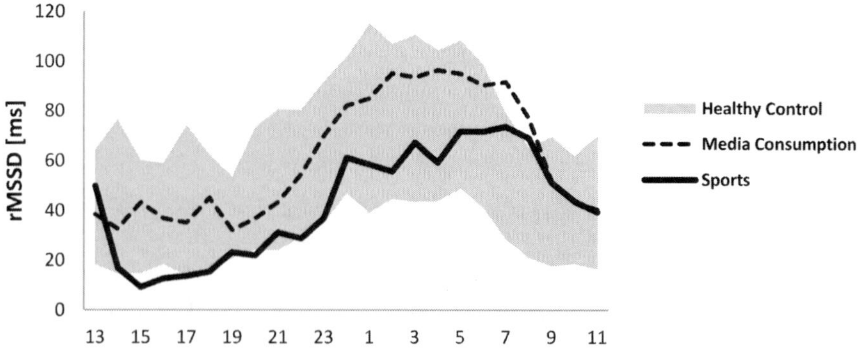


Figure 5.2. Vagus recovery after sports between 14:00 and 16:00 (compared to media consumption) in the 7 children with the lowest HRV.

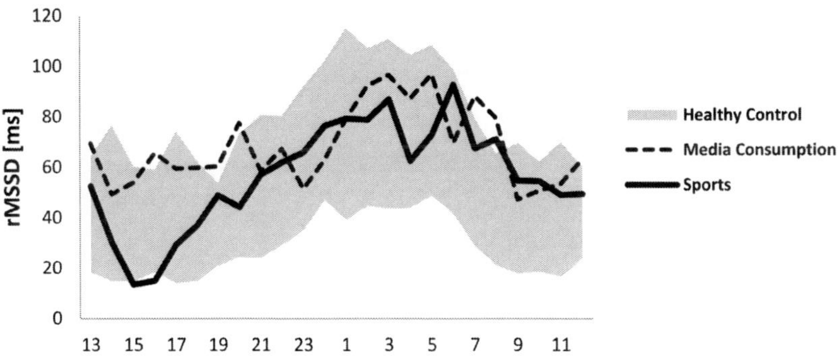


Figure 5.3. Vagus recovery after sports between 14:00 and 16:00 (compared to media consumption) in the 7 children with the highest HRV.

Chapter 6

# HRV in Children with Heart Disease

Heart failure and sudden cardiac death are the final common path of nearly all heart disease in childhood. Heart failure remains the main cause of death in children with heart disease. In USA and Europe hospital mortality of children with heart failure is about 7%, nearly twice as high as in adults. "Congenital heart diseases account for more life years lost than leukemia and asthma combined and acquired heart disease of childhood are increasing contributors to childhood morbidities".... However, "pediatric cardiovascular clinical trials rarely focused on specific congenital malformations and more commonly focused on diseases and conditions typically considered high impact adult cardiovascular diseases" (Hill et al., 2014). Accordingly, children don't have access to the progress of medical heart failure therapy and are only treated with digoxin and diuretics for more than 50 years. As most drugs used for the treatment of cardiovascular disease are modulators of the autonomic nervous system I would like to discuss the role of the autonomic nervous system in heart disease in childhood.

## 6.1. HRV in Children with Congenital Heart Disease Prior to Surgery

The prevalence of heart failure in infants with congenital heart disease, mainly due to large left to right shunt, is as high as 20%. In this subgroup of patients ventricular systolic function is, unlike in adults with heart failure, usually preserved. But infants commonly develop symptoms like tachypnea, failure to thrive, and hepatomegaly. The morphology of congenital heart defects is the cause of the well-known hemodynamic disturbances, but cannot explain clinical symptoms like tachypnea and failure to thrive. The neurohormonal hypothesis, regarding heart failure not only as a hemodynamic derangement but also as a neurohormonal disorder, may be valid in infants with left-to-right shunts (Buchhorn et al., 2001a). Infants with clinical signs of heart failure demonstrated severe hormonal changes consistent with activation of the renin-angiotension-aldosterone- and sympathetic nervous system. Elevated norepinephrine levels and reduced HRV are evidence for sympathetic activation in infants with tachypnea. We could demonstrate that autonomic imbalance in infants with congenital heart disease can be measured by reduced HRV with evidence of a high diagnostic sensitivity. Reduced HRV is related to elevated norepinephrine levels (Figure 6.1) but only the global HRV (SDNN) seems to be related to the clinical signs of heart failure in infants with left to right shunts indicated by the Ross Score (Figure 6.2 and 6.3). In summary, HRV represents a noninvasive parameter that is reduced in infants with congenital heart disease depending on the severity of heart failure and neurohumoral activation.

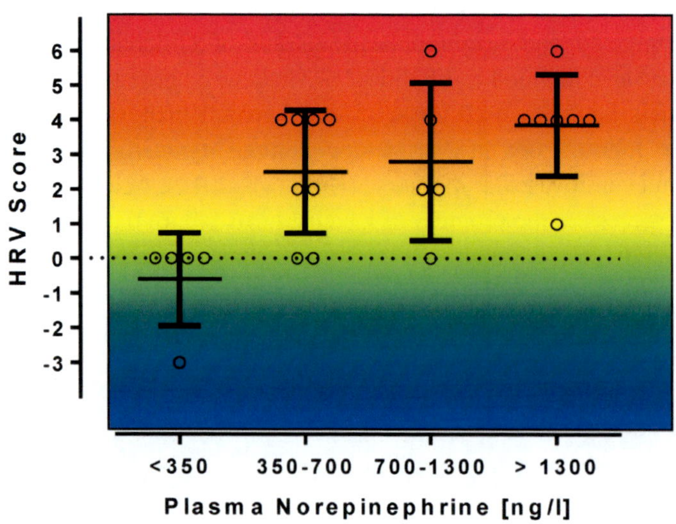


Figure 6.1. HRV Score and norepinephrine levels in 29 infants with heart failure.

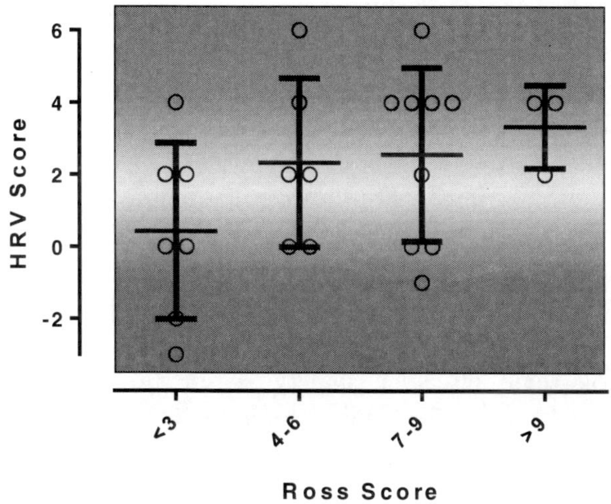


Figure 6.2. HRV Score and a clinical heart failure Score (Ross Score) in infants with heart failure.

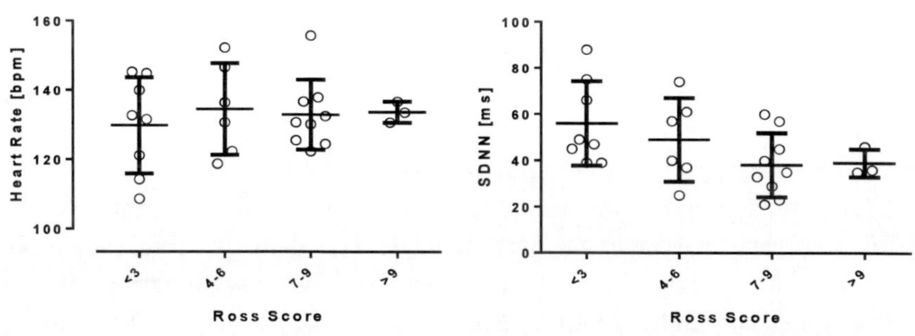


Figure 6.3. HRV Score and a clinical heart failure Score (Ross Score) in infants with heart failure.

## 6.2. HRV after Surgery of Congenital Heart Defects

Several authors have shown reduced HRV in children after surgery of congenital heart defects. Their explanation for postoperative autonomic dysfunction after cardiac surgery includes heart failure and/or surgery-related damage to cardiac autonomic nerve fibers. Central sympathetic and parasympathetic heart nerves pass along the posteromedial surface of the superior vena cava, the right atrium, and both the ascending aorta and main pulmonary artery (Janes et al., 1986). I agree with the authors who found no correlation of autonomic dysfunction with norepinephrine levels and heart failure indicated by natriuretic peptides or ventricular function (Ohuchi et al., 2011) (Figure 6.4.). It is important to realize that reduced HRV is related to markers of sustained ventricular tachycardia and sudden cardiac death (Davos et al., 2002b). However our more sophisticated analysis does not support the idea that HRV is related with the number and complexity of surgical procedures (Ohuchi et al., 2004;Ohuchi et al., 2011). HRV in our group is not related to the complexity of cardiac surgery measured by the Aristotle Score (Lacour-Gayet & Clarke, 2005) (Figure 6.5) or previous palliative procedures (Figure 6.6.). We measure the best HRV Scores in children who were operated on as neonates or after the age of 6 years (Figure 6.7). There may be a trend to better HRV Scores in children operated on within the last 10 years (Figure 6.8).

Although postoperative HRV doesn't seem to be related to heart failure as indicated by the biomarker NT-Pro BNP (Figure 6.4) we measured the highest maximal oxygen uptake during spiroergometry (Figure 6.9) in patients with a normal HRV Scores between (-1) and (+2). There is a trend to a more pronounced reduction of HRV in patients after surgery of left-to-right shunts compared to surgery for cyanotic defects (Figure 6.10).

In summary, autonomic dysfunction only occur in some patients after cardiac surgery of congenital heart defects. The damage of the autonomic nervous system is not related to the complexity of cardiac surgery as recently demonstrated in children with transposition of the great arteries after arterial switch operation (Doksoz et al., 2014). These patients have not decreased levels of time and frequency HRV in the mid-term follow-up period despite highly complex surgery as neonates. We speculate that preoperative damage of the autonomic nervous system due to heart failure in infancy may be the reason for a lifelong autonomic dysfunction (see chapter autonomic programming). I am convinced that "stress" prevention in infants with congenital heart disease by early corrective surgery like shown in children after arterial switch operation and - if not possible - with propranolol treatment of heart failure is necessary to prevent autonomic dysfunction. An effective preoperative heart failure therapy with propranolol may be the reason that longtime HRV after cardiac surgery seems to be improved in my patients after the year 2000 (Buchhorn & Ross, 2014b).

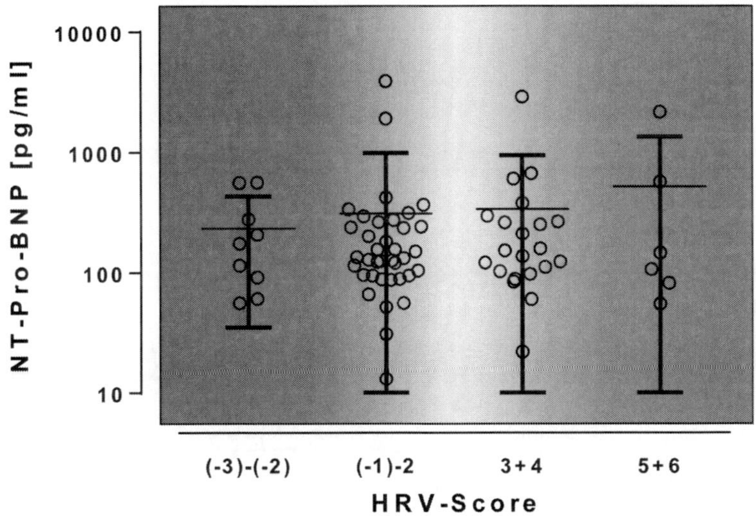


Figure 6.4. HRV Score and NT-Pro-BNP levels late after surgery for congenital heart disease.

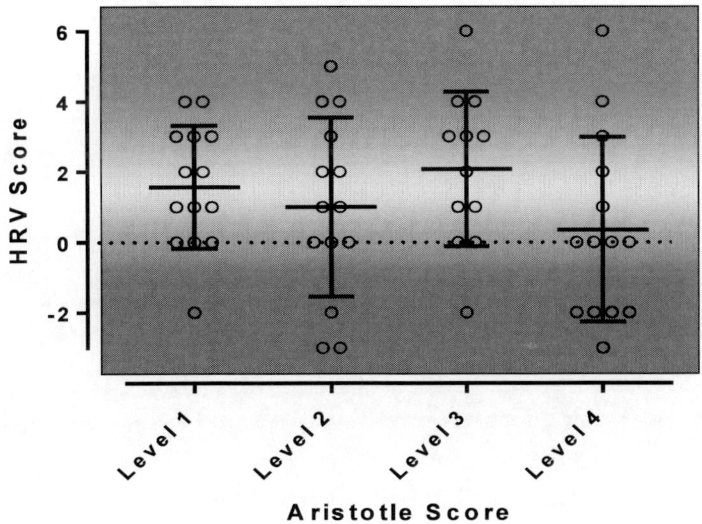


Figure 6.5. HRV Score and complexity of cardiac surgery measured by the Aristotle Score.

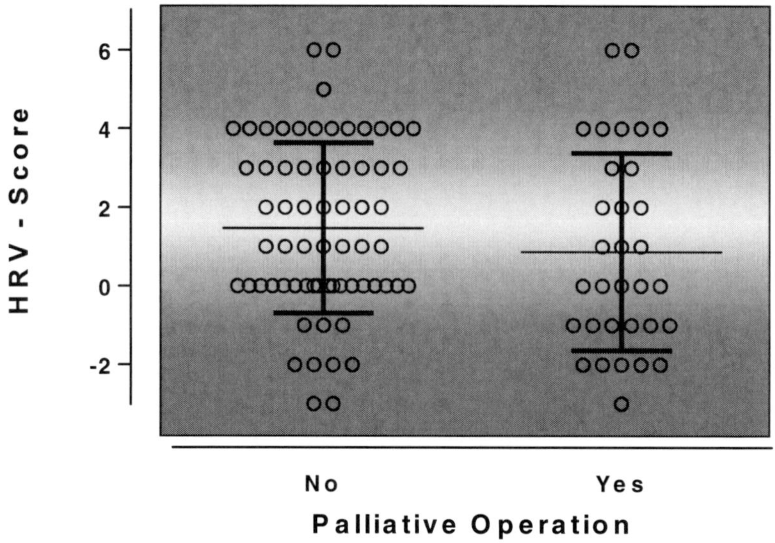


Figure 6.6. HRV Score and palliative procedures in patients with congenital heart defects.

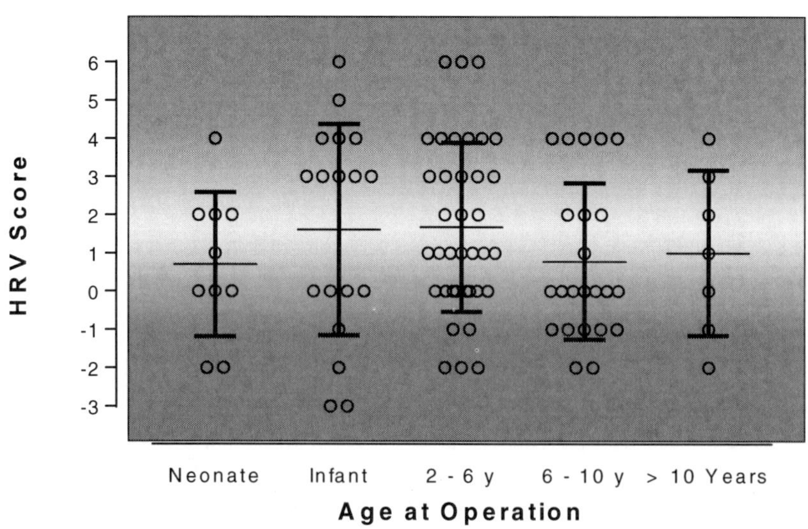


Figure 6.7. HRV Score and age at operation in patients with congenital heart defects.

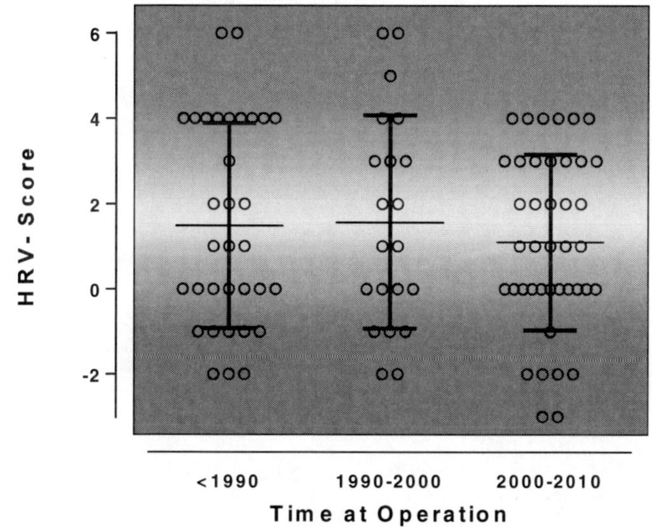


Figure 6.8. HRV Score and time at operation in patients with congenital heart defects.

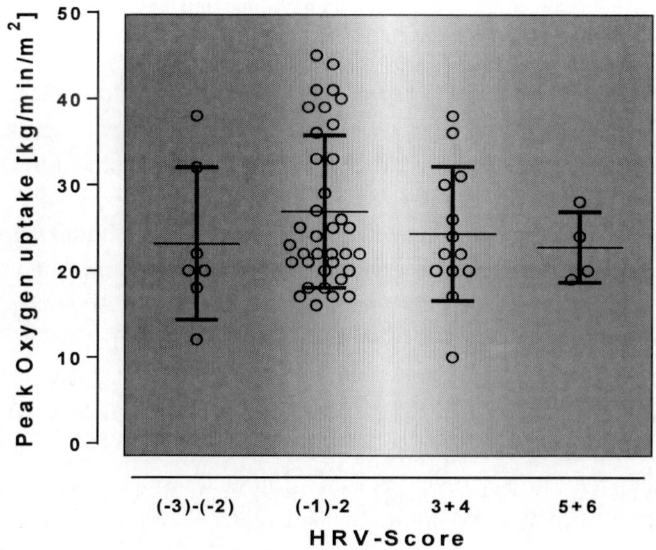


Figure 6.9. HRV Score and maximal oxygen uptake late after surgery for congenital heart disease.

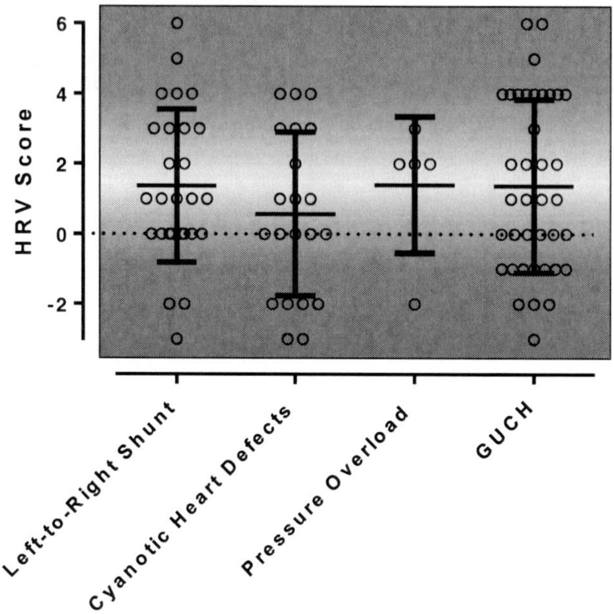


Figure 6.10. HRV Score and basic hemodynamic in patients with congenital heart defect (GUCH=Grown up with congenital heart defect).

The complex situation of the so called "denervated" heart is illustrated in a 27 year old mean after corrective surgery of Fallot's tetralogy (Figure 6.11). At the first visit, 6 years ago, he had been treated with digoxin for nearly his whole life and he had accumulated several risk factors: obesity with a BMI of 31.6 kg/sqm, smoking, and reduced physical capacity with a maximal oxygen uptake of 20.8 ml/kg/min at spiroergometry. Digoxin was terminated but I was not able to convince him for a change of his detrimental life style. 2 years later he lost nearly 20 kg bodyweight during an endocarditis lenta. Despite successful antibiotic therapy he developed aortic valve insufficiency and had low heart rate variability (SDNN = 75ms) treated with 47.5mg Metoprolol succinate. HRV improved but worsened again after the patient stopped medical therapy of his own accord. Initiated by omega-3-fatty acid supplementation he decided for a fundamental change of his life style by eating fish and performing daily sports. Again he reduce his body mass index to 28.3 kg/sqm and without any medical therapy his HRV significantly improved to normal values (SDNN=185 ms). This case clearly demonstartes that HRV of the so called denervated heart clearly benefit from beta-blockers and life style changes as well.

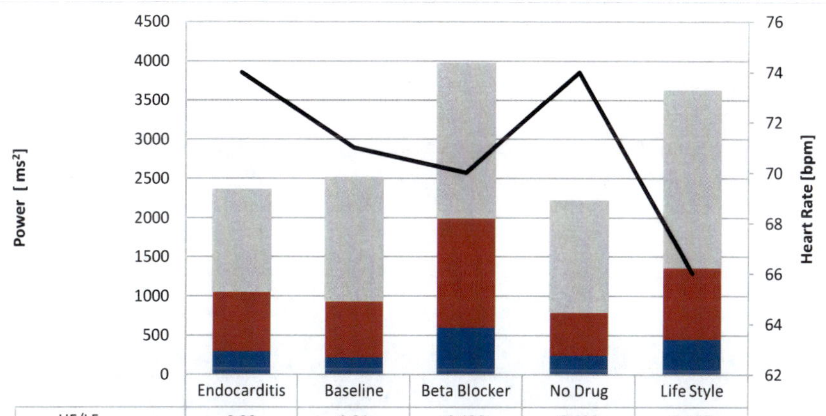


| | Endocarditis | Baseline | Beta Blocker | No Drug | Life Style |
|---|---|---|---|---|---|
| HF/LF | 0,39 | 0,31 | 0,428 | 0,429 | 0,488 |
| VLF | 1302 | 1572 | 1962 | 1414 | 2255 |
| LF | 763 | 719 | 1405 | 563 | 920 |
| HF | 296 | 224 | 601 | 241 | 449 |
| Heart Rate [bpm] | 74 | 71 | 70 | 74 | 66 |

Figure 6.11. Late follow up of a 27 years old man after corrective surgery of Fallot's tetralogy. There is an impressive improvement of HRV after a life style change despite aortic and pulmonary valve insufficiency.

## 6.3. HRV in Children with Left Ventricular Dysfunction

A small part of children with heart disease suffer from heart failure due to left ventricular dysfunction due to myocarditis or cardiomyopathies. In these cases we found good correlations between the severity of heart failure, NT-Pro-BNP levels and the HRV Score. As shown in Figure 6.12. we use HRV monitoring together with NT-Pro-BNP monitoring to control medical therapy with angiotensin converting enzyme inhibitors, beta-blockers and diuretics. In this boy with end stage heart failure due to Duchenne cardiomyopathy up-titration of carvedilol was only possible after an immunadsorption therapy. With this treatment, we used the immunadsorption as "bridge to beta-blocker therapy" , the boy has now survived a further 3 years with a very good quality of life. Using HRV monitoring we were able to control a further new approach to treat heart failure with coenzyme Q (Mortensen et al., 2014) when at the age of 17.5 years his heart failure worsened again.

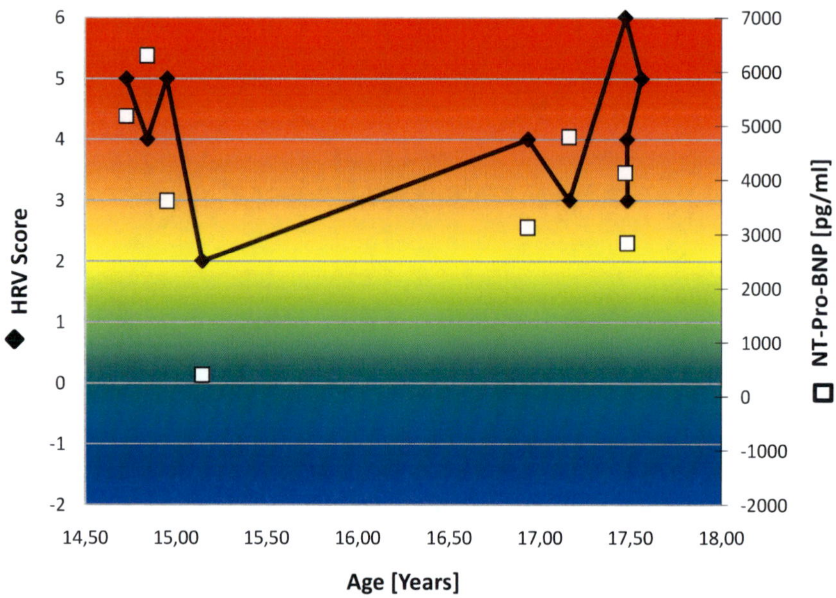


Figure 6.12. HRV Score in a boy with end-stage heart failure due to Duchenne cardiomyopathy. He received immunoadsorption therapy and carvedilol at the age of 15 years and Carvedilol dose escalation and Coenzyme Q supplementation at the age of 17.5 years.

## 6.4. HRV and Arrhythmias

The autonomic nervous system plays an important role in sudden cardiac death (Vaseghi & Shivkumar, 2008). Twenty-four-hour Holter recordings after post myocardial infarction in adult patients showed that depressed HRV was a significant predictor of mortality after adjusting for clinical and demographic features, including ejection fraction. HRV is also reduced in survivors of sudden cardiac death not associated with coronary artery disease (Fei et al., 1994). It is noticeable that adults with rMSSD values below 15 ms irrespective of cardiovascular risks have a significantly higher risk of sudden cardiac death. Sudden infant death syndrome may also be related to autonomic dysfunction where infants have rMSSD values below 15ms. This statement is nevertheless based on mere pathophysiological speculations deduced from widely accepted theories on how the autonomous nervous system relates to sudden cardiac death.

### 6.4.1. Arrhythmias in Children with Autonomic Dysfunction

The fact that children without heart disease suffer from arrhythmias caused by autonomic dysfunction is widely ignored by paediatricians. Over the years our discussions have focused on the cardiovascular side effects of stimulants in children with attention deficit disorder. Most of these publications have been based on theoretical speculations according to the proarrhythmogenic effects agents closely related members to the class of sympathomimetic amines (Nissen, 2006). Unfortunately, only a few publications report about clinically measured cardiovascular data in these patients. The reason for these uncertainties is, that in contrast to adults, sudden death occurs rarely in the general pediatric population and the modeling to predict the incidence of sudden cardiac arrest in healthy children has been compared to searching for a needle in a haystack. For cardiac risk assessment there is no doubt that history and physical examination is important, but ambiguities in current screening recommendations with respect to electrocardiogram assessment show the lack of sufficient surrogate measurements.

Our studies about autonomic imbalance in children with ADHD show evidence for an increased cardiovascular risk by the disorder itself independently from medical treatment - indicated by reduced heart rate variability and ventricular arrhythmias (Buchhorn et al., 2012a;Buchhorn et al., 2012b). By Holter electrocardiogram analysis we observed a remarkably high incidence of ventricular arrhythmias in 9 of 100 children with attention deficit disorder (Buchhorn & Christian, 2013b). All these children had ventricular parasystole – four of them with an accelerated idioventricular rhythm. A significant circadian rhythm of premature ventricular contractions in seven children and the effect of standing and exercise clearly indicate the influence of the autonomic nervous system. In these children hourly analysis of circadian rhythm showed a highly significant correlation between premature ventricular contractions and vagal tone indicated by the heart rate variability parameter rMSSD (Figure 6.13. ; $r = -0.83$; $p<0.001$). The ventricular arrhythmia seems to have been unaffected in seven children who received methylphenidate prior to diagnosis and decreased during metoprolol treatment in two children. We found an impressive reduction of premature ventricular contractions in three children who received omega 3 fatty acids supplementation. These results are in accordance with the higher cardiovascular risk in untreated patients with attention deficit disorders in the large observational studies as well as the higher cardiovascular risk of adults with psychiatric disorders (Cooper et al., 2011a). A better pathophysiological understanding of heart - brain - interactions in children with autonomic disorders will improve diagnostics and opens new therapeutic options for these children.

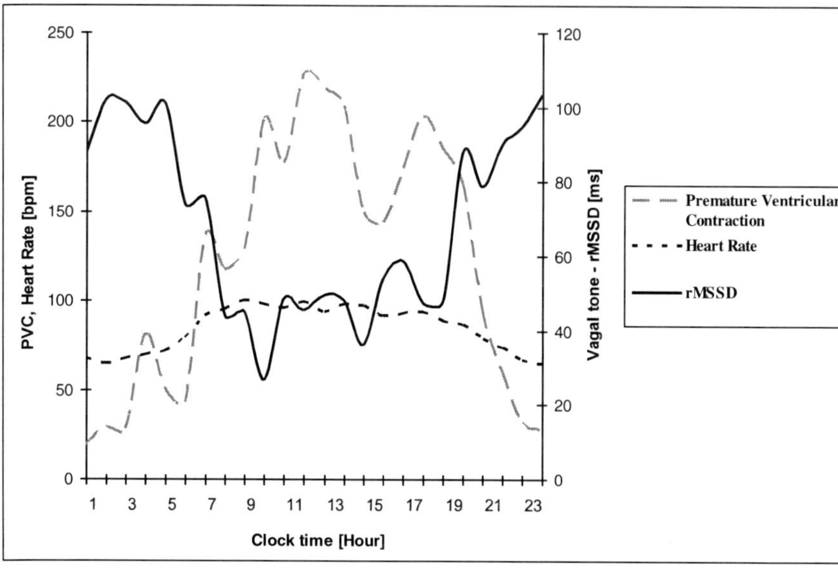


Figure 6.13. Mean hourly values of premature ventricular contractions, heart rate and the heart rate variability paramter rMSSD which represents vagal tone in 7 children with ADHD and arrhythmias. Premature ventricular contractions significantly correlate with heart rate (r=0.77; p<0.0001) and rMSSD (r=-0.83; p<0.0001).

## 6.4.2. Arrhythmias in Children with Heart Disease

30 to 50% heart failure patients die a sudden cardiac death as compared with progressive pump failure or other complications. The annual incidence of sudden cardiac death in patients with heart failure was 1.8% (Fan et al., 2014). Reduced HRV is a proven predictor of sudden cardiac death in patients with heart failure (Wu et al., 2014) and arrhythmogenic right ventricular dysplasia (Battipaglia et al., 2012). Our data particularly indicates that most of all heart rate correlate with arrhythmias in a patient with cardiomyopathy (Figure 6.14 and 6.15).

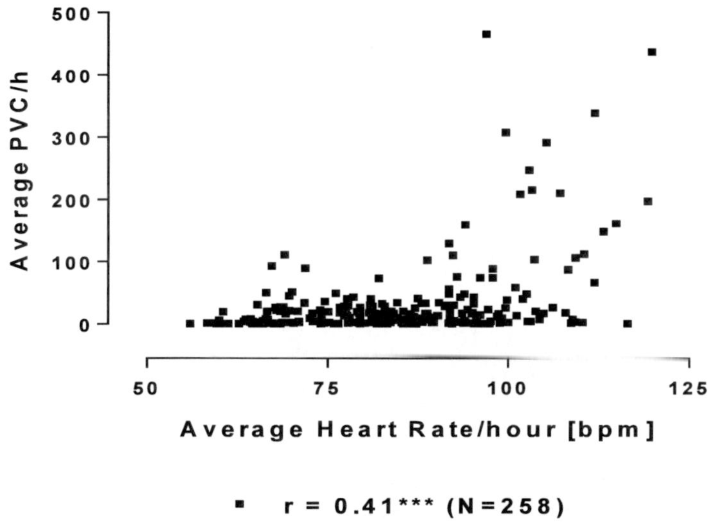


Figure 6.14. Correlation of hourly premature ventricular contraction (PVC) and mean heart rate in the boy with Duchenne cardiomyopathy within 3.5 years.

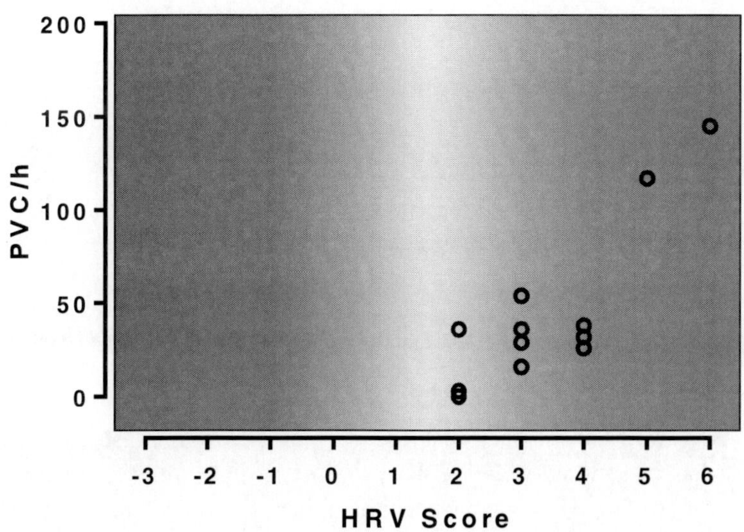


Figure 6.15. HRV Score of twelve 24 hour Holter ECG's and the average of premature ventricular contraction (PVC) per hour in a boy with end stage heart failure within 3.5 years.

In contrast, premature ventricular contractions occur in patients with heart defects independent from HRV (Figure 6.16). However in these patients reduced HRV was related to sustained ventricular tachycardia and sudden cardiac death (Folino et al., 2004) (Davos et al., 2002a).

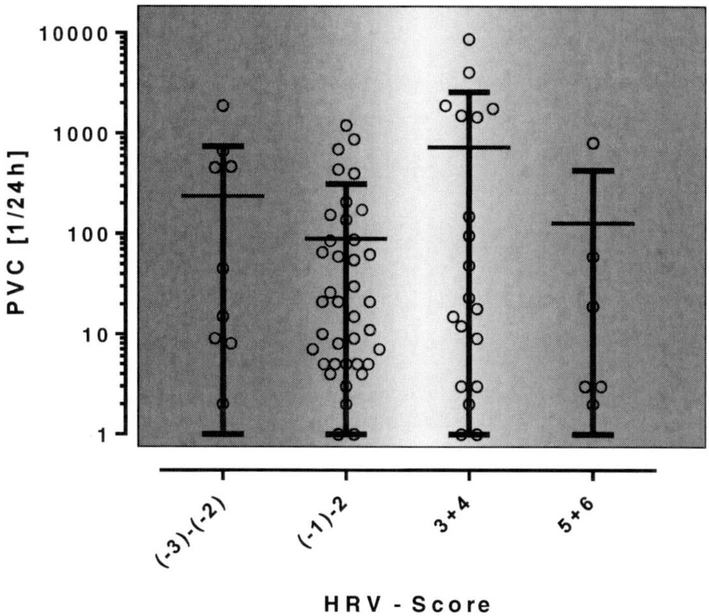


Figure 6.16. HRV Score of the 24 hour Holter ECG and the average number of premature ventricular contractions in patient with congenital heart defects.

## 6.4.3. HRV and in Children with Paroxysmal Supraventricular Tachycardia

It is a well-known fact that the risk of paroxysmal supraventricular tachycardias in children with WPW syndrome is high in the first year of life and adulthood. There is high evidence that this risk is related to the maturation of the autonomic nervous system as illustrated in the Figure 6.17. Improving HRV by omega-3-fatty acids may be beneficial in this patient group.

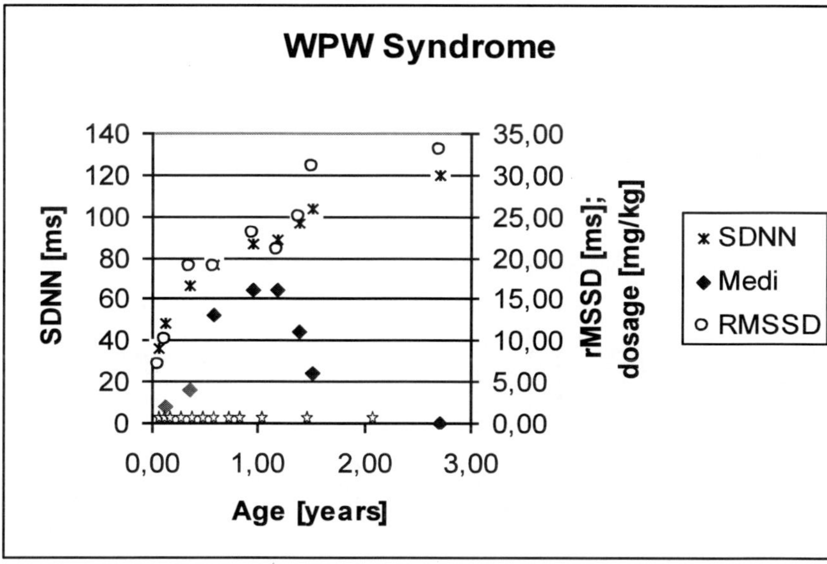


Figure 6.17. Escalation and de-escalation of drug therapy with Propranolol (◆) and Propafenon (◆) in a boy with WPW Syndrome. Paroxysmal supraventricular tachycardias (☆) disappear and need no further antiarrhytmic drug therapy after physiological vagal maturation indicated by the increase of rMSSD and global HRV (SDNN).

The immediate HRV changes at the onset of a paroxysmal supraventricular tachycardia is shown in the Figure 6.18. Surprisingly there is a phasic increase of total power in all frequencies. This figure demonstrates a spontaneous, unperceived and untreated tachycardia at sleep and also demonstrates the phasic decrease of this "autonomic storm" at the end of the second tachycardia. The tachycardia can be recognized by the complete loss of total power when such a reentry tachycardia has the same RR-Interval.

Vagal activity is indicated by HF to LF ratio and rMSSD in Figure 6.19 which shows a steep increase of vagal activity just before the onset of the tachycardia that may indicate a parasympathetic trigger of this arrhythmia. The indication of a parasympathetic trigger is in accordance with previously published data from 90 adults who showed a vagal prevalence in the minutes before the onset of paroxysmal atrial fibrillation (Vincenti et al., 2006).

Again the autonomic nervous system provides us with major challenge: On one hand the vagus protects us against arrhythmias on the other hand sudden increase of vagal activity may induce a paroxysmal tachycardia.

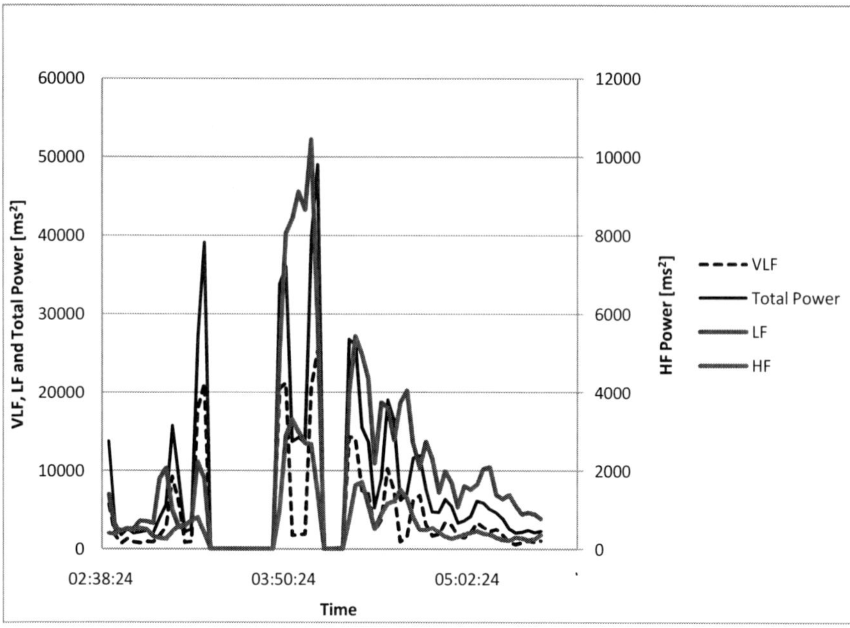


Figure 6.18. Onset of a paroxysmal supraventricular tachycardia in a 16 years old boy at night while sleeping (3:08 and 4:48).

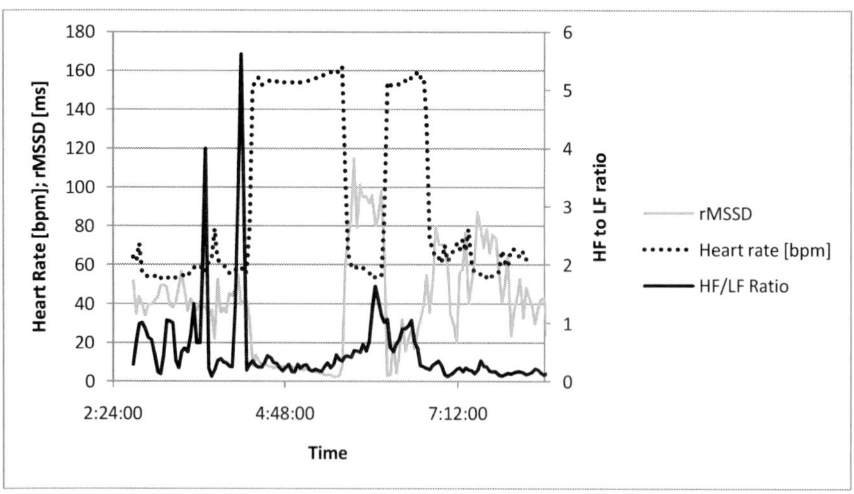


Figure 6.19. HF to LF ratio and rMSSD just before the onset of a paroxysmal supraventricular tachycardia in a 16 years old boy that may indicate a parasympathetic trigger of this arrhythmia.

# 6.5. Hypertension and HRV

The Framingham Study showed that low HRV predicts arterial hypertension (Jelinek et al., 2013). These results are confirmed in a study with young adults from India (Pal et al., 2012d). This data further showed a relationship between HRV, hypertension and body mass index (Pal et al., 2012b). However the increase of blood pressure in healthy children from US and Germany is not only related to a higher body mass index (Wabitsch et al., 2002). We recently published findings demonstrating that a vagus shift in healthy children from today may explain the slight increase of blood pressure which impacts cardiovascular prognosis (De Bock et al., 2013).

A further recently published case of the first successful renal sympathetic denervation in a child after resection of aortic coarctation (Buchhorn et al., 2014) demonstrates the interplay between the kidney and the autonomous nervous system. After renal sympathetic denervation we observed not only lower blood pressures but also a breakthrough of sympathetic dominance indicated by the HRV Score (Figure 6.20.).

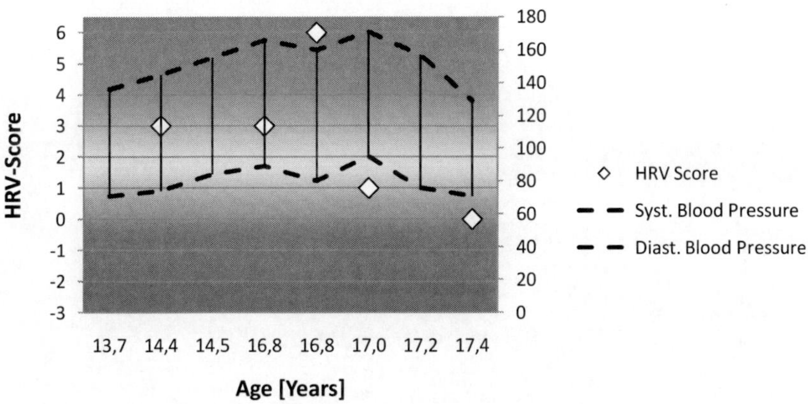


Figure 6.20. Blood pressure and HRV Score after a successful renal sympathetic denervation at an age of 17.0 years after resection of aortic coarctation.

*Chapter 7*

# HRV and Growth

The inverse association between height and ischemic heart disease has been studied extensively over the last six decades, from the first report in 1951 to a recent metaanalysis of 52 studies (Paajanen et al., 2010). In summary adults in the shortest height category were at approximately 50% higher risk of ischemic heart disease morbidity and mortality than tall individuals. Patients with low birth weight (in the stricter sense "small for gestational age" = SGA) (Risnes et al., 2011) and growth hormone deficiency (=GHD) (Capalbo et al., 2013) are the focus of current investigations. If these children are candidates for growth hormone therapy our knowledge about the effect of this therapy on cardiovascular risk has to be improved. Autonomic imbalance may be the final common pathway to increased morbidity and mortality in cardiovascular disease. Global heart rate variability (HRV) indicated by the parameter SDNN (standard deviation of normal RR-intervals) may be used to assess autonomic imbalances, diseases and mortality in adults (Thayer et al., 2010a; Jelinek et al., 2013) and children (Zhou et al., 2012). Sympathetic activity indicated by low rMSSD and pNN50 values have been associated with a wide range of conditions including cardiovascular disease. We systematically used HRV analysis for cardiovascular risk stratification in children with growth failure:

With the exception of children with constitutional growth delay, all other children with short stature show a trend to sympathetic dominance (Figure 7.1.). This trend is more pronounced in children with growth hormone deficiency and in children with growth failure due to heart disease. Children with growth failure due to intrauterine growth retardation show an intermediate result. In detail global heart rate variability (SDNN) seems to be normal in children with short stature up to the age of 8 years and is diminished in older short children with and without growth hormone therapy (Figure 7.2.). A similar trend could be shown for the vagal parameter rMSSD (Figure 7.3.). According to this observation the statistics for the whole group only show significant higher heart rates and lower SDNN in the untreated children with short stature.

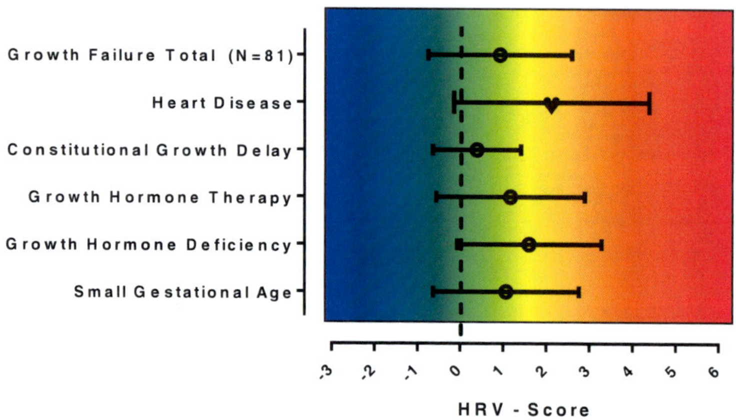


Figure 7.1. HRV Score and growth failure due to heart disease, constitutional growth delay, small gestational age and growth hormone deficiency.

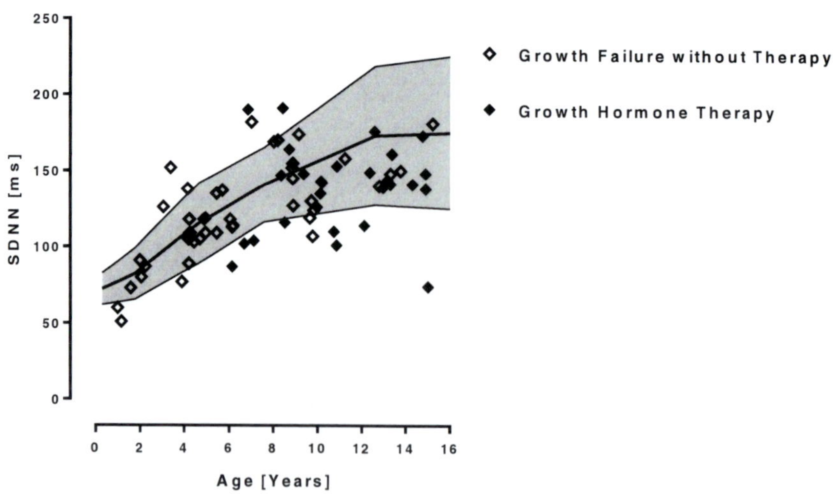


Figure 7.2. Gobal HRV indicated by the parameter SDNN in children with growth failure with and without growth hormone therapy compared to healthy children (gray curve mean ± one standard deviation).

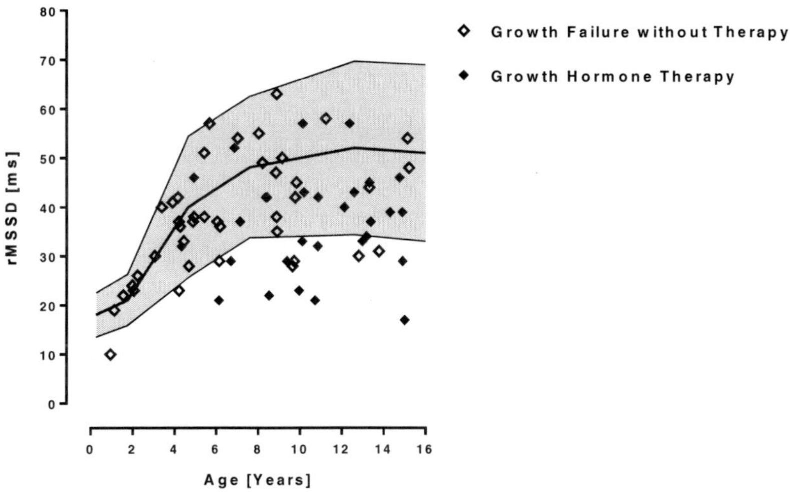


Figure 7.3. Vagal activity indicated by the parameter rMSSD in children with growth failure with and without growth hormone therapy compared to healthy children (gray curve mean ± one standard deviation).

**Table 7.1. HRV in children with growth failure with and without growth hormone therapy**

| | All Children 1-16 years | | | | |
|---|---|---|---|---|---|
| Parameter | Healthy Control (N=121; ♀:60/♂:61) | Growth Failure (N=30; ♀:15/♂:15) | | Growth Hormone Therapy (N=30; ♀:14/♂:16) | |
| | Mean±SD | Mean±SD | p-value | Mean±SD | p-value |
| Age | 8.9 ± 4.4 | 6.3 ± 3.6 | 0.001 | 10.8 ± 3.7 | 0.034 |
| Height Percentile [%] | 48 ± 27 | 1,2 ± 1 | 0,000 | 6,6 ± 6,8 | 0,000 |
| Weight Percentile [%] | 43 ± 24 | 7 ± 13 | 0,000 | 12 ± 11 | 0,000 |
| BMI Percentile [%] | 41 ± 25 | 33 ± 24 | 0,27 | 34 ± 25 | 0,73 |
| Heart Rate [bpm] | 90 ± 15 | 99 ± 11 | 0.000 | 89 ± 10 | 0.70 |
| Heart Rate Day | 100 ± 20 | 111 ± 11 | 0,007 | 99 ± 11 | 0,83 |
| Heart Rate Night | 76 ± 17 | 84 ± 9 | 0,001 | 77 ± 10 | 0,86 |
| SDNN [ms] | 149 ± 51 | 118 ± 29 | 0.000 | 137 ± 30 | 0.10 |
| rMSSD [ms] | 46 ± 18 | 42 ± 14 | 0.43 | 43 ± 17 | 0.53 |
| Total Power | 4957 ± 3029 | 3737 ± 1708 | 0,01 | 4931 ± 2300 | 0,97 |
| VLF | 2839 ± 2241 | 2016 ± 1101 | 0,10 | 2828 ± 1643 | 0,98 |
| LF | 1303 ± 709 | 1008 ± 507 | 0,024 | 1361 ± 697 | 0,69 |
| HF | 731 ± 353 | 613 ± 271 | 0,14 | 656 ± 244 | 0,28 |
| HF/LF | 0,61 ± 0,22 | 0,66 ± 0,24 | 0,31 | 0,54 ± 0,20 | 0,10 |

Our results are in accordance with W. Aziz et al. (Aziz et al., 2012) who found significantly reduced HRV in 70 children with a birthweight below 2500g at an age between 9 and 10 years. In contrast HRV parameters were significantly enhanced in 15 healthy adults aged 20 to 30 years with low birthweight <2500g published by G. Weitz et al.(Weitz et al., 2013). However this study only includes SGA patients with catch up growth. HRV was reduced in eleven untreated adults with GHD at mean age 50.4 ± 10.7 years (Leong et al., 2000).

*Chapter 8*

# Effects of Pharmacotherapy on HRV

## 8.1. Effect of Clonidin on HRV in Children with Growth Failure

Recently a blunted response to the clonidine growth hormone stimulation test was found to be associated with unfavourable cardiovascular risk factor profile in childhood cancer survivors (Petryk et al., 2013). For a better understanding of the link between human height and cardiovascular risk we analyse HRV in children with a height below the third percentile, who attend our outpatient clinic. We do not only analyse HRV under baseline conditions (see chapter 7) but also during a routine clonidine growth hormone stimulation test (N=56).

The $\alpha_2$-adrenoreceptor agonist clonidine is a powerful inhibitor of the sympathetic autonomic system. It stimulates growth hormone (GH) release in both children and adults. It has been used to test for GH deficiency in children and to assess central $\alpha_2$-adrenoreceptor function in adults in order to determine the pathophysiological basis and to confirm diagnosis in neurological diseases with autonomic failure. The secretion of growth hormone is regulated by a complex neuroendocrine control system based on the balance between two hypothalamic neurohormones: growth hormone-releasing hormone, exerting a stimulative influence upon growth hormone secretion and somatostatin, which has an inhibitory effect. In summary Clonidine release growth hormone effect is based on its action upon $\alpha$2-adrenoceptors.

Patients with short stature and suspected growth hormone deficiency spent a day in our clinic for a routine testing with Clonidine. Clonidine stimulation was performed with an oral dose of 0.15 $mg/m^2$ body surface area.

As expected, clonidine had an overall sympatholytic effect indicated by lower LF and HF/LF values and leads to vagal activation indicated by higher rMSSD (table 8.1). However at the clonidine test we observed vagal activation only in children with constitutional growth delay (CGD) and in small gestational age (SGA) children (table 8.1). Notably all children with growth hormone deficiency (GHD) showed no changes in HRV after clonidine administration which would suggest an underlying hypothalamic problem (Figure 8.1). These results indicate that at least these children with GHD may have a genuine subsensitivity to the $\alpha_2$-adrenoreceptor and that the growth hormone deficiency in this case is not caused by a pituitary problem. Additionally, the small group of children with SGA without catch up growth showed no sympathetic inhibition indicated by the HF to LF ratio by clonidine (Figure 8.2) and there also seems to be higher rMSSD values at night in the SGA group independent from clonidine given at 9:00 in the morning (table 8.1, Figure 8.1).

In contrast to constitutional growth retardation, children with idiopathic isolated growth hormone deficiency and small gestational age seems to display attributes of a "stress" disease independent from actual psychosocial stress due to their short stature, which is equal in these groups. A functional $\alpha_2$-adrenoreceptor subsensitivity mediating clonidine induced growth hormone secretion has been described in Wistar rats after chronic hydrocortisone treatment (Aulakh et al., 1994). A link between diurnal cortisol rhythms and child growth was shown in a longitudinal study exploring the life history consequences of hypothalamic pituitary axis in children of a foraging society in the Bolivian Amazon (Nyberg et al., 2012b). We speculate that hypothalamic $\alpha_2$-adrenoreceptor subsensitivity as shown in children with GHD and probably in SGA is the missing link between early programming of the hypothalamic pituitary axis, growth failure and enhanced cardiovascular risk (Reynolds et al., 2001;Reynolds et al., 2013). Understanding of these mechanisms whereby early stressors may be transmitted from mother to foetus will not only improve our knowledge of normal foetal and neonatal development but will also help identify novel pathways for early interventions. Our simple modification of the clonidine growth hormone stimulation test by simultaneous HRV analysis will help us to examine the hypothalamic $\alpha2$-adrenoceptors function in different somatic and psychosomatic diseases.

**Table 8.1. Vagal activation indicated by the parameter rMSSD due to clonidine in children with constitutional growth delay (CGD), small gestational age (SGA) and growth hormone deficiency (GHD)**

| | Baseline | | rMSSD [ms] during Clonidine Test at 9:00 T- test versus age matched baseline controls | | | | | | | | |
|---|---|---|---|---|---|---|---|---|---|---|---|
| | Healthy Control N = 36 | | CGD N = 36 | | | GHD N = 14 | | | SGA N = 6 | | |
| Time | MW | SD | MW | SD | p-value | MW | SD | p-Wert | MW | SD | p-value |
| 8 | 36.2 | 20.7 | 37.4 | 19.1 | 0.80 | 39.5 | 27.4 | 0.43 | 33.0 | 12.7 | 0.644 |
| 9 | 31.2 | 17.8 | 34.9 | 20.0 | 0.42 | 32.2 | 18.7 | 0.52 | 32.1 | 11.8 | 0.421 |
| 10 | 29.0 | 15.5 | 44.7 | 19.2 | <0.001 | 34.8 | 18.4 | 0.29 | 61.9 | 26.0 | 0.015 |
| 11 | 28.5 | 18.3 | 53.3 | 23.5 | <0.001 | 43.5 | 25.9 | 0.08 | 80.5 | 36.8 | 0.012 |
| 12 | 29.5 | 18.1 | 48.4 | 24.8 | 0.001 | 28.7 | 18.1 | 0.30 | 47.3 | 35.4 | 0.284 |
| 13 | 30.1 | 14.4 | 42.2 | 30.6 | 0.041 | 43.8 | 34.4 | 0.33 | 63.1 | 44.2 | 0.115 |
| 14 | 28.7 | 12.9 | 47.9 | 29.6 | 0.001 | 41.4 | 27.7 | 0.67 | 57.2 | 21.9 | 0.028 |
| 15 | 28.5 | 12.8 | 38.7 | 23.3 | 0.026 | 38.2 | 22.6 | 0.78 | 62.2 | 35.7 | 0.142 |
| 16 | 27.6 | 12.0 | 37.6 | 26.6 | 0.045 | 37.2 | 22.0 | 0.88 | 51.7 | 37.5 | 0.171 |
| 17 | 27.1 | 12.1 | 38.2 | 23.8 | 0.016 | 33.6 | 25.5 | 0.79 | 49.4 | 20.5 | 0.014 |
| 18 | 29.1 | 15.6 | 31.7 | 21.6 | 0.56 | 36.1 | 19.9 | 0.87 | 32.3 | 12.0 | 0.142 |
| 19 | 29.7 | 17.3 | 32.6 | 16.0 | 0.47 | 35.6 | 18.0 | 0.79 | 50.5 | 28.9 | 0.310 |
| 20 | 35.6 | 18.9 | 42.4 | 21.2 | 0.16 | 43.4 | 18.5 | 0.24 | 78.5 | 25.4 | 0.007 |
| 21 | 48.2 | 22.8 | 55.9 | 33.7 | 0.26 | 57.3 | 32.3 | 0.54 | 108.7 | 44.0 | 0.009 |
| 22 | 55.1 | 24.7 | 63.0 | 36.6 | 0.29 | 63.7 | 23.4 | 0.84 | 127.7 | 42.0 | 0.006 |
| 23 | 62.2 | 26.1 | 68.5 | 28.6 | 0.33 | 70.0 | 35.2 | 0.53 | 137.1 | 39.9 | 0.001 |
| 24 | 62.8 | 25.1 | 72.9 | 31.5 | 0.14 | 81.4 | 37.2 | 0.52 | 145.1 | 76.3 | 0.019 |
| 1 | 58.9 | 29.0 | 70.2 | 36.9 | 0.16 | 76.2 | 38.4 | 0.86 | 95.9 | 29.1 | 0.009 |
| 2 | 62.1 | 30.4 | 68.1 | 35.0 | 0.44 | 71.7 | 45.2 | 0.51 | 114.0 | 29.9 | 0.040 |
| 3 | 67.1 | 34.6 | 67.3 | 33.4 | 0.98 | 78.4 | 31.3 | 0.77 | 93.1 | 32.6 | 0.026 |
| 4 | 69.8 | 28.8 | 70.8 | 31.1 | 0.88 | 68.2 | 28.6 | 0.31 | 99.8 | 73.1 | 0.296 |
| 5 | 59.5 | 25.8 | 58.0 | 27.3 | 0.81 | 60.4 | 29.2 | 0.20 | 75.2 | 16.3 | 0.125 |
| 6 | 60.2 | 28.2 | 55.3 | 30.0 | 0.48 | 53.5 | 20.3 | 0.17 | 87.3 | 40.0 | 0.173 |
| 7 | 44.8 | 23.2 | 43.9 | 21.6 | 0.87 | 32.4 | 12.8 | 0.06 | 53.0 | 29.7 | 0.823 |

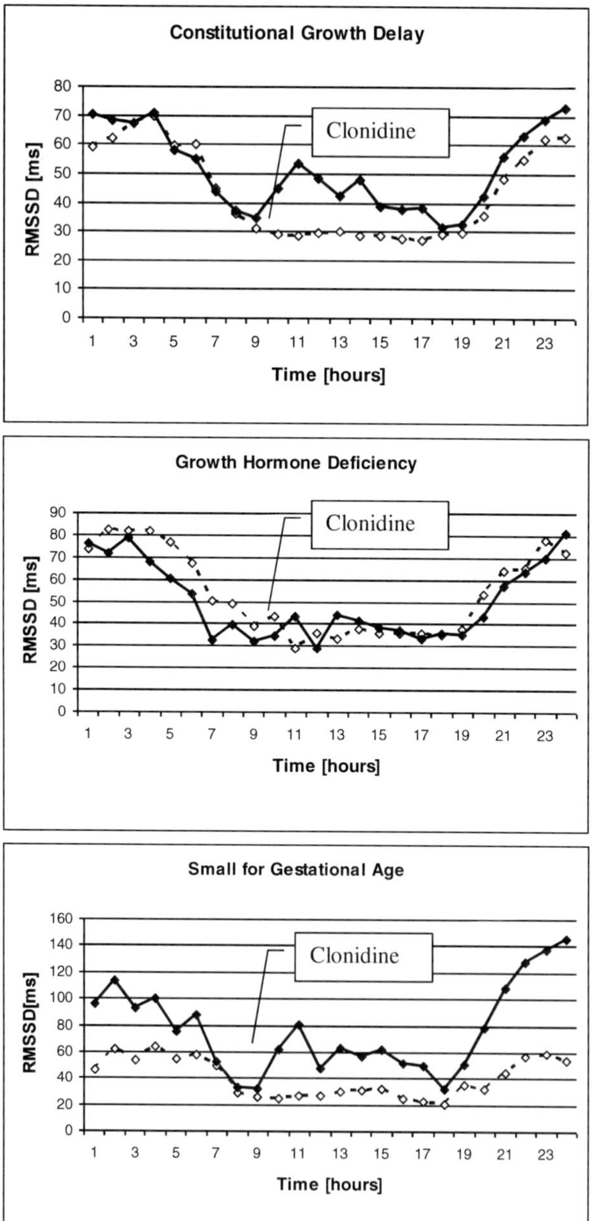


Figure 8.1. Effect of clonidine given at 9:00 on the vagal parameter rMSSD in children with growth failure due to constitutional growth delay, growth hormone deficiency and small gestational age (♦) compared to baseline data of an age matched healthy control group (◊).

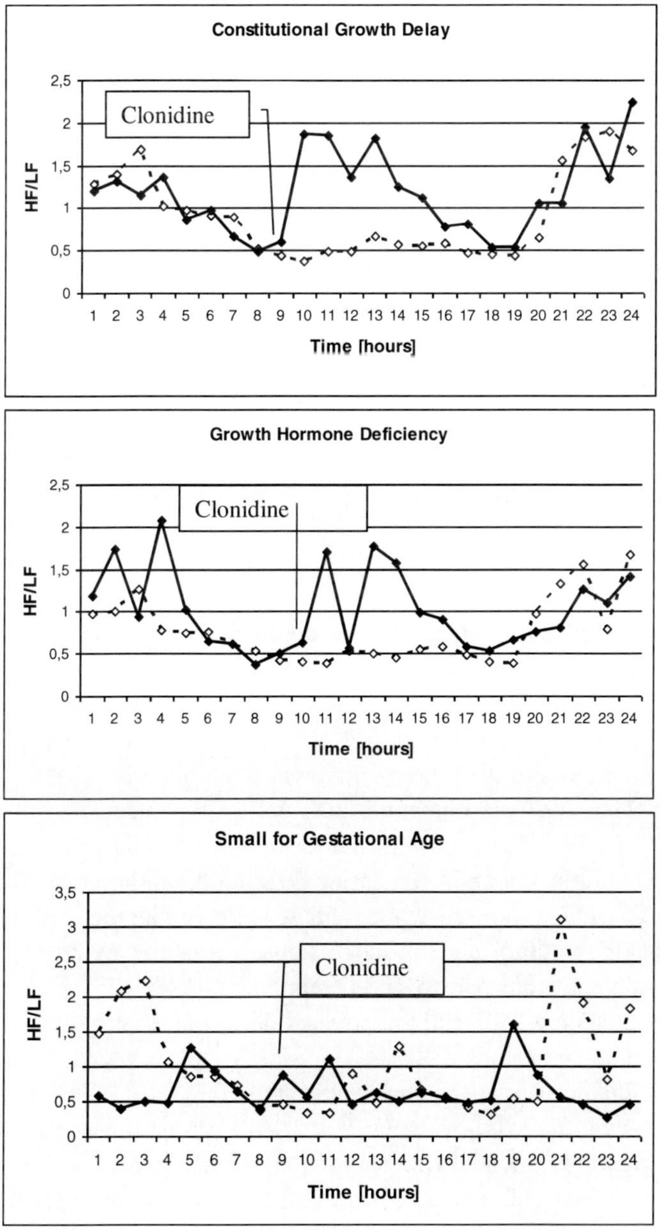


Figure 8.2. Effect of clonidine given at 9:00 on the autonomic balance indicated by the parameter HF/LF in children with growth failure due to constitutional growth delay, growth hormone deficiency and small gestational age (♦) compared to baseline data of an age matched healthy control group (◊).

As shown in children with GHD we are able to detect $\alpha_2$-adrenoreceptor subsensitivity long time before global HRV is reduced. The test will be able to analyse the hypothalamic α2-adrenoceptors function not only in patient groups but also on an individual base if we use 24 hours HRV a day before the clonidine test as individual baseline.

## 8.2. Effect of Growth Hormone Therapy on HRV

The effect of growth hormone replacement therapy on HRV in adults with GHD showed contradicting results (Tanriverdi et al., 2005; Leong et al., 2001). In these patients growth hormone therapy induced an autonomic switch to sympathetic dominance indicated by a reduced SDNN and higher LF to HF ratios. These effects clearly indicate a negative cardiovascular effect and not the positive effect which was projected by the authors.

Little is known of the long-term health of children treated with growth hormone in childhood. SAGhE is a European consortium aimed at adressing this question. A preliminary report of the French SAGhE study showed an increase in mortality of 6928 children due to disease of the circulatory system (SMR 3.07, 95% CI 1.4-5.83) (Carel et al., 2012). This excess mortality is related to the highest growth hormone doses >50 μg/kg/day (SMR 2.94, 95% CI 1.22-7.07) as well as to height at initiation of treatment < - 3 SDS (SMR 2.31, 95% CI 0.96-5.59). Consolidated results of the complete SAGhE study were expected to be disseminated during 2013 (still waiting) but it is unlikely that this high volume project will be able to differentiate the expected excess cardiovascular mortality due to short stature, from the treatment effect of growth hormone therapy. However, this important question has to be answered for approximately 40000 children treated in Europe and several hundred thousand in the world.

In this situation our HRV data as indicated in Figure 7.2. and 7.3. are very helpful to predict the cardiovascular risk in children with growth failure with respect to growth hormone therapy in each individual case.

Nearly 12% of children with heart defects develop growth failure below the third percentile at an age of 36 months (Daymont et al., 2013a). The most important risk factor is heart failure during infancy. Moreover elevated BNP-values in infants due to heart failure are related to final height and mental disorders(Ravishankar et al., 2013). Improving the therapy of heart failure in infancy most of all by early corrective surgery and/or medical therapy with beta-blockers will improve the prevalence of growth failure and mental outcome in children with heart disease. The effect of growth hormone therapy in children with heart failure was investigated in a prospective study published in *Pediatrics* (McElhinney et al., 2004). Of the 8! study patients, 2 children needed heart transplantation because of worsening heart failure. Despite this inconclusive outcome, the authors saw "some beneficial hemodynamic effects". Unfortunately there are no attempts to measure neurohormonal parameters as shown in adults with heart failure treated with growth hormone (Acevedo et al., 2003).

One of my cases, a 10 years old boy with severe heart failure due to dilated cardiomyopathy and growth failure due to growth hormone deficiency (-4.2 SDS) received a low dose of 0.2 mg/kg growth hormone. His implanted biventricular pacemaker monitored his volume state and showed a steep increase of volume load shortly after introducing the growth hormone therapy as shown in Figure 8.4. Adequate diuresis was only successful by addition of thiazides to high dose loop diuretics to achieve a sequential blockade of the nephron. However NT-BNP further increase (Figure 8.3) and the boy developed renal failure and had to be listed for heart transplantation. Taken together, "living" is more important than "growing" and children with heart failure should not be treated with growth hormone as recommended in *Pediatrics*.

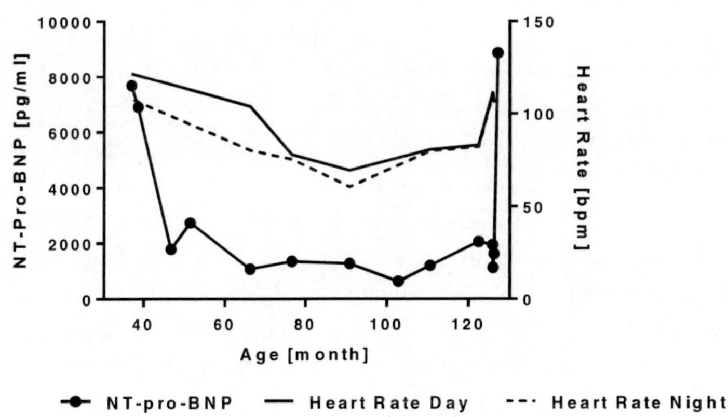


Figure 8.3. Worsening heart failure in a 10 years old boy who was treated with growth hormone at an age of 120 month. There is an increase of heart rate after starting growth hormone despite the ongoing beta blockade therapy with carvedilol.

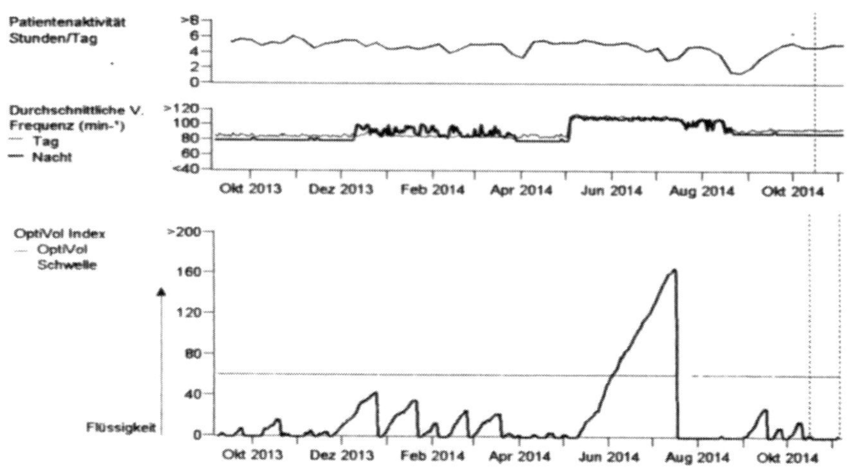


Figure 8.4. Volume state of an 10 years old boy with heart failure measured by the implanted biventricular pacemaker (OptiVol™). After introduction of growth hormone therapy in June 2014 he developed volume retention treated with addition of thiazides to high dose loop diuretics to achieve a sequential nephron blockade. One week after the successful treatment of volume retention he developed renal failure.

# 8.3. Effect of Beta-blockers on HRV in Children

Neurohormonal inhibition is the foundation of modern heart failure management. Beta-blocker therapy has led to a decrease in mortality due to their effects on heart failure and sudden cardiac death. The benefits of beta-blockers in patients with heart failure due to reduced ejection fraction seem to be a class effect as no statistical evidence from current trials supports the superiority of any 1 agent over the others. The beneficial effect is primarily due to the beta receptor blockade and its lowering of the heart rate. There have been concerns that beta-blockers may be deleterious in severe or NYHA Class IV heart failure, and in heart failure associated with diabetes mellitus or pulmonary obstruction. But as indicated in table 8.2, these meta-analyses provide evidence that the same survival benefit may be seen from beta-blockers in severe heart failure patients with and without diabetes mellitus, or pulmonary obstruction (Buchhorn & Ross, 2014a).

To investigate the effect of beta-blockers on HRV in infants with congenital heart disease we analyzed three patients groups comparable in age and hemodynamic relevance of their cardiac lesions. All infants needed cardiac surgery within the first year of life. The 'Digoxin/Diuretics' and

**Table 8.2. Results of the beta-blocker trials in adult heart failure**

| Metaanalysis Beta-Blockers for Heart Failure | | | | Mortality | | |
|---|---|---|---|---|---|---|
| Subgroup Analysis | Trials | Patients | Beta-Blocker Recommendation | OR | CI | Significance |
| Heart Failure | 21 | 23122 | Yes | 0.69 | 0.56 - 0.8 | <0.001 |
| Sudden Death | 30 | 24779 | Yes | 0.69 | 0.62 – 0.77 | < 0.00001 |
| Heart Rate | 17 | 17831 | Yes | 0.82 | 0.71 – 0.94 per 5 bpm ↓ | < 0.001 |
| HFp(reserved) EF | 12 | 21206 | Yes | 0.91 | 0.87-0.95 | < 0.001 |
| NYHA IV | OPTIMIZE-HF | 2373 | Yes | 0.6 | 0.37 – 0.99 | 0.044 |
| Diabetes Mellitus | 6 | 13129 (3230) | Yes | 0.72 | 0.65 – 0.79 | <0.001 |
| Pulmonary Obstruction | | 722 | Yes | Lung functional test | | |
| FEV 1 | 10 | 141 | | -0.42% | -3.74 – 2.91 | n.s. |

'Propranolol' patients groups are from the CHF-PRO-INFANT trial (Buchhorn et al., 2001b). Patients of the 'CHD Control' group were excluded from this trial because of lesser signs of heart failure and a Ross Score below 7 points. The norepinephrine and renin levels in 'Digoxin/Diuretics' and 'Propranolol' groups were markedly increased in contrast to the 'CHD Control' group.

**Table 8.3. Analysis of heart rate variability in infants with heart failure due to left-to-right shunts**

| | Healthy Control (N = 70) | CHD Control (N=12) | Digoxin/ Diuretics (N = 14) | Propranolol (N = 9) |
|---|---|---|---|---|
| **Baseline characteristics** | | | | |
| Age [month] | 2,1 ± 2,7 | 4,8 ± 3,1 | 2,6 ± 1,9 | 3,7 ± 1,7 |
| Ross Score | | 2,7 ± 2,5 | 8,0 ± 2,4 | 2,9 ± 1,8 |
| Norepinephrine [ng/l] | 646 ± 238 | 560 ± 247 | 1156 ± 705 | 916 ± 652 |
| Mean RR [msec] | 437 ± 40 | 469 ± 45 | 445 ± 31 | 511 ± 48** |
| SDNN [ms] | 57,4 ± 18,9 | 56,5 ± 16,5 | 37,4 ± 11,7** | 45,0 ± 18,7 |
| pNN50 [%] | 2,15 ± 2,76 | 4,58 ± 4,65 | 1,56 ± 2,48 | 8 ± 12,9 |
| rMSSD [ms] | 22,1 ± 8,7 | 20,2 ± 8,6 | 14,7 ± 6,9** | 23,1 ± 14,8 |

Plus-minus values are means ± SD
Results of student-t-test between patient group and healthy control: * p = 0,001 - 0,01; ** p < 0,001

Heart rate in the 'Digoxin/Diuretics' group was higher in comparison to the 'Propranolol' and 'CHD Control' group which were not significantly different to the 'Healthy Control' (Tab 8.3). Nearly all HRV parameters under 'Digoxin/Diuretics' were significantly reduced but in contrast, we observed normal time domain measures in the 'CHD Control' and the 'Propranolol' group.

In conclusion HRV represents a noninvasive parameter that is reduced in infants with congenital heart disease depending on the severity of heart failure and neurohumoral activation. Propranolol but not digoxin therapy effectively reduced the perceived autonomic imbalance in infants with severe heart failure due to congenital heart disease (Buchhorn et al., 2002c;Buchhorn & McConnell, 2014).

Our so called BB-BUCH trial investigated beta blockade with Bisoprolol on asymptomatic or mildly symptomatic young adults with right ventricular dysfunction secondary to repaired tetralogy of Fallot with residual pulmonary regurgitation and/or stenosis (Norozi et al., 2007). There seems to be no beneficial effect on brain natriuretic peptide levels and peak oxygen uptake and despite a significant reduction of average heart rates, HRV did not improve in 13 study patients (table 8.4.).

**Table 8.4. Analysis of heart rate variability in young adults with tetralogy of Fallot**

| | Beta-blocker (N=13) | | Placebo (N=20) | |
|---|---|---|---|---|
| | Start | End | Start | End |
| Baseline characteristics | | | | |
| Age [years] | 28.8 ± 9.8 | | 32.2 ± 9.2 | |
| BNP [pg/ml] | 206 ± 95 | 341±250* | 173 ± 128 | 160 ± 86 |
| Peak Oxygen Uptake | 22 ± 2 | 23 ± 4 | 21 ± 2 | 22 ± 2 |
| Heart rate [bpm] | 71 ± 9 | 64 ± 9* | 76 ± 8 | 76 ± 11 |
| Time domain | | | | |
| SDNN [ms] | 137 ± 39 | 131 ± 29 | 119 ± 28 | 119 ± 34 |
| rMSSD [ms] | 41 ± 19 | 46 ± 14 | 32 ± 19 | 35 ± 19 |
| sNN50 [N] | 16 ± 14 | 19 ± 12 | 12 ± 13 | 12 ± 12 |

Plus-minus values are means ± SD

Results of student-t-test between patient group and healthy control: * p = < 0,01; ** p < 0,001.

The effect of the beta-blocker carvedilol on HRV in 34 children with dilated cardiomyopathies was recently published (Oflaz et al., 2013). Table 8.5. shows the significant improvement of the clinical heart failure score together with lower heart rates and an improvement of heart rate variability indicated by SDNN and rMSSD.

**Table 8.5. Effect of carvedilol on HRV in 34 children with dilated cardiomyopathies (Oflaz et al., 2013)**

| | Baseline | Carvedilol | p-value |
|---|---|---|---|
| Ross Score | 6 (5-10) | 3(2-7) | 0.030 |
| Heart Rate [bpm] | 114 ± 23 | 83 ± 21 | 0.008 |
| SDNN [ms] | 98.7 ± 35.6 | 133.4 ± 39.2 | 0.002 |
| rMSSD [ms] | 23.6 ± 15.2 | 32.6 ± 19.4 | 0.008 |
| PVC [n/h] | 62.4 ± 19.6 | 48.6 ± 17.1 | 0.016 |

Recently we investigated the effect of beta blockade on HRV from adolescents without heart defects. These 10 patients received Metoprolol or Propanolol to treat arrhythmias or headache. Administering the doses in the morning, we found a significant heart rate reduction during the day without any effect on heart rate at night but little effect on HRV (table 8.6/Figure 8.5). Taken together, although beta-blockers reduce heart rate in all patients, beta-blockers only improve HRV in patients with reduced HRV (for example due to heart failure) but not in patients with normal HRV.

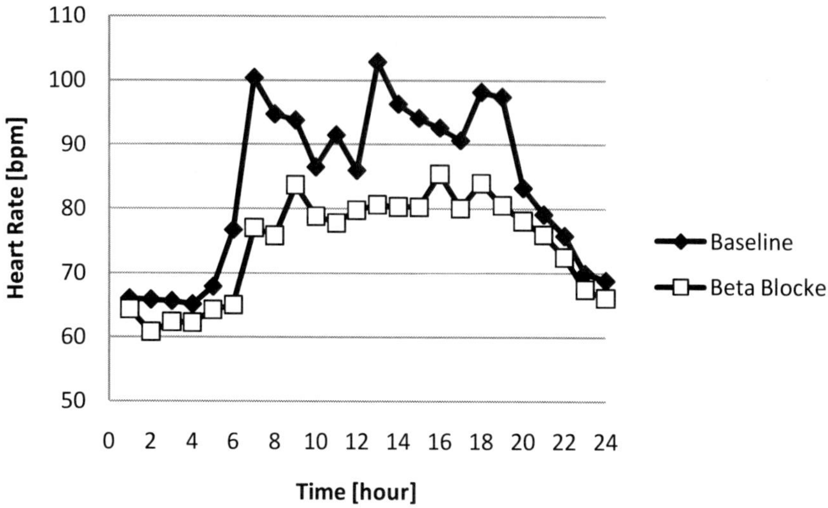


Figure 8.5. Effect of a beta-blocker on heart rate in children without heart disease.

**Table 8.6. Effect of a beta-blocker on HRV in children without heart disease**

| | Baseline | | Beta-Blocker Therapy | | |
|---|---|---|---|---|---|
| | N= 10 | | | | |
| Gender | 6♀ : 4♂ | | | | |
| | Mean | +/- SD | Mean | +/- SD | p-value |
| Age | 13.2 | 4.3 | | | |
| Heart rate [bpm] | 81 | 10 | 74*** | 12 | 0.0003 |
| Heart rate day [bpm] | 90 | 10 | 80**** | 13 | <0.0001 |
| Heart rate night [bpm] | 69 | 9 | 65* | 11 | 0.0372 |
| SDNN [ms] | 154 | 36 | 161 | 57 | 0.5839 |
| rMSSD [ms] | 43 | 22 | 50* | 25 | 0.0183 |
| TP 24h | 5736 | 3570 | 7726 | 5879 | 0.1256 |
| VLF 24h | 3618 | 2488 | 5206 | 4464 | 0.1486 |
| LF 24h | 1367 | 712 | 1675 | 1089 | 0.1095 |
| HF 24h | 689 | 450 | 779 | 467 | 0.2828 |
| HF/LF 24h | 0.48 | 0.13 | 0.48 | 0.13 | 0.9538 |

After propranolol treatment of an infant with severe heart failure due to haemangiomatosis in 2002 in our department, beta-blocker therapy of children with haemangioma became a very popular therapy (Lou et al., 2014) due to its effect of haemangioma regression. This therapy seems to be safe but the effect of propranolol given in the vulnerable period of autonomic programming in infancy is unclear. If our concept of autonomic programming (chapter 9) is right this therapy will have consequences on height and neurodevelopment.

## 8.4. Effect of Methylphenidate on HRV in Children with Attention Deficit Disorder

Potential side effects of stimulants are currently the focus of scientific discussions. This focus has been intensified by the higher number of prescriptions. An extensive number of studies support efficacy and tolerability of stimulants, however, in 2006, the United States Food and Drug Administration added a black box warning that stimulants may cause serious cardiovascular effects like high blood pressure and even sudden death. The assumption that stimulant treated ADHD patients are at higher risk for sudden death was based on the proarrhythmogenic effects of these agents, which are closely related members to the class of sympathomimetic amines. A general contraindication was stated for children with known serious heart rhythm abnormalities, or other severe cardiac problems, which may increase their vulnerability to the sympathomimetic effects of stimulants (http://www.fda.gov/ohrms/dockets/ac/oc06.htm). However, a recently published large retrospective cohort study showed no evidence that current use of an attention deficit disorder drug was associated with an increased risk of serious cardiovascular events in children (Cooper et al., 2011b) or young and middle-aged adults (Habel et al., 2011).

Our data now indicates that untreated children who suffer from ADHD show significant changes in HRV which predominantly reflect diminished vagal tone, a well-known risk factor of sudden cardiac death in adults. In our pilot study methylphenidate treatment improved HRV and a simple 24 hour analysis of heart rate could clarify the current misunderstanding that stimulants increase heart rate. We could only find higher rates within 2 hours after methylphenidate was given in the morning (Figure 8.6). Later in the day, the heart rate in methylphenidate treated children was higher compared to the healthy control group but lower than the heart rate of untreated ADHD patients. This surprising effect is explained by the effect on vagal activity (sNN50 or rMSSD) which is clearly improved in methylphenidate treated

ADHD patients (Figure 8.7). It is an interesting pharmacological phenomenon that the sympathomimetic action of MPH on the autonomous nervous system within the first half of the day causes the most prominent changes in HRV during the night, when MPH has probably already been metabolized.

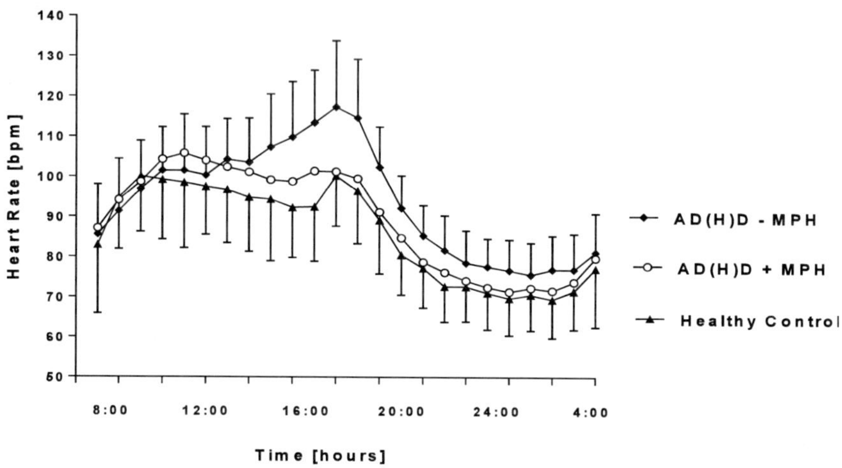


Figure 8.6. Effect of methylphenidate (MPH) given early in the morning on heart rate in children with ADHD.

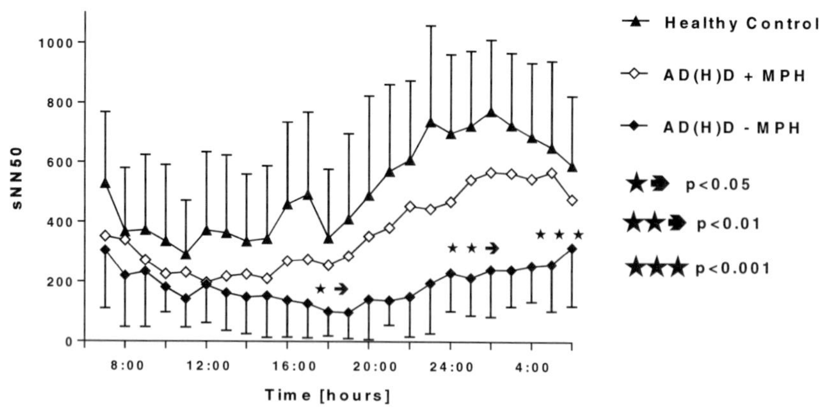


Figure 8.7. Effect of methylphenidate (MPH) on vagal activity indicated by the parameter sNN50 in children with ADHD.

However, recently published data from Denmark in children with ADHD (n=8300) showed an increased risk of a cardiovascular event during stimulant treatment (adjusted HR=2.20 [2.15-2.24]), with a complex time-dependent dose-response relationship (Dalsgaard et al., 2014).

## 8.5. Effect of Caffeine on HRV

The autonomic effect of methylphenidate in children with ADHD is comparable with effect of caffeine in adults measured with same methodological approach by Richardson et al. (Richardson et al., 2004). It is very interesting that caffeine, the most often used stimulant with long tradition in humans, has the autonomic effects as methylphenidate which is the most often used stimulant in children.

Chapter 9

# Autonomic Programming

Genome-wide Single Nucleotide Polymorphism analyses have identified genomic variants associated with adult human height. However, these only explain 10% of human height (≈ 3 cm) (Simeone & Alberti, 2014). There are speculations that even 90% may be explainable by epigenetic.

Early life stress has a programming effect (Spencer, 2013) on the hypothalamus-pituitary-axis (HPA) and seems to be related to growth failure (Nyberg et al., 2012a). Stunting is considered to be the best global indicator of children's well-being, and growth impairment has both short and long-term consequences. There is strong evidence that stunting is associated with delayed mental development, and that there is a relationship between impaired growth status and both poor school performance and reduced intellectual achievement. Starvation in infancy due to problems of breast feeding (Figure 9.1) cause the same drop in heart rate and in HRV as shown in adolescents with anorexia nervosa. As recently published, this autonomic damage in infants with failure to thrive goes along with enhanced NT-Pro-BNP levels and is comparable to data measured in infants with severe heart failure (Manhardt et al., 2010). All these infants are at risk of a lifelong autonomic dysfunction causing growth failure, mental disorders and enhanced cardiovascular risk.

Our model how early life stress may cause stunting, enhanced cardiovascular risk and impaired neurodevelopment is illustrated in Figure 9.2. In the centre of our reflections stands the hypothalamic α2-adrenoceptor who seems to play an important role in the regulation of the hpothalamus-pituitary-axis and the autonomic nervous system. A subsensitivity of hypothalamic α2-adrenoceptor , like shown in children with growth hormone deficiency and small gestational age, may explain many symptoms of this children including stunting, enhanced cardiovascular risk and neurocognitive disorders. “Exposure of the fetus to increased levels of glucocorticoids, resulting from maternal stress or treatment with synthetic glucocorticoids, can lead to long-term 'programming' of hypothalamic-pituitary-adrenal function and behaviours.

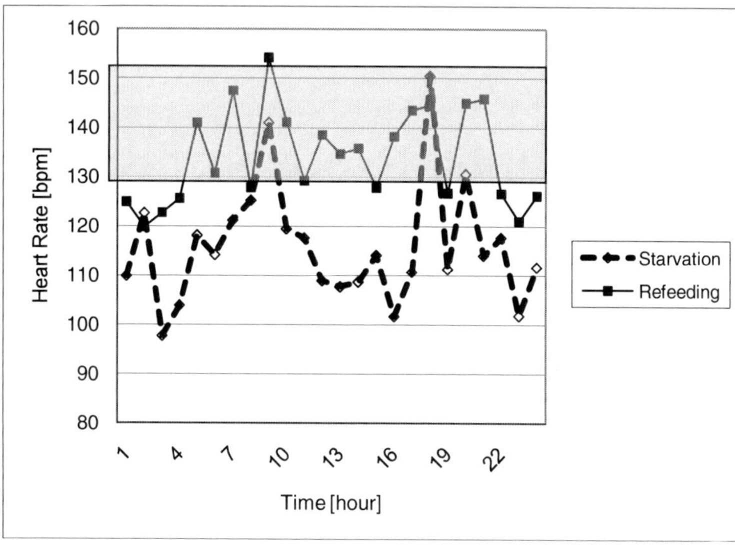


Figure 9.1. Circadian heart rate of infants with starvation during breast feeding and 2 weeks later after re-feeding with formula nutrition compared to healthy infants (gray bar).

Growing evidence indicates that they can exert powerful effects on the epigenome, including on DNA methylation, histone acetylation and microRNA, to influence gene expression. Such influences probably represent a critical component of the 'programming' process, and might be partly responsible for the transgenerational effects of antenatal glucocorticoid exposure on neurologic, cardiovascular and metabolic function.” (Moisiadis & Matthews, 2014).

However epigenetic changes and α2-adrenoceptor function are only measured in animal models. With our methodological approach we are able to measure HRV as an indicator for early life stress and α2-adrenoceptor function as shown in chapter 8.1. in an everyday setting.

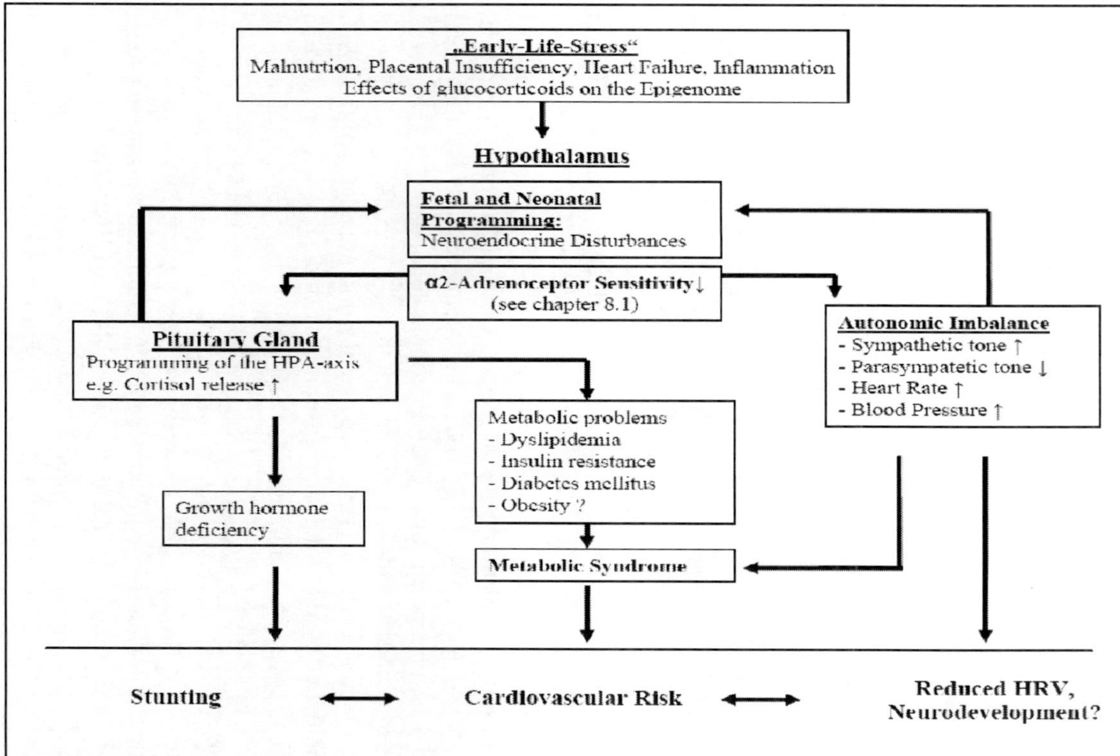


Figure 9.2. Model of autonomic/neuroendocrine programming by early life stress (Doctor’s thesis S. Meint/R. Buchhorn).

When searching for the best model of early life stress and fetal programming there is a large number of publications about intrauterine growth restriction. However, heart failure in infancy is one of the most prominent stressful life events and that is best indicated by elevated norepinephrine levels and highly reduced heart rate variability in 24 hour ECG monitoring (Buchhorn et al., 2001c;Buchhorn et al., 2002b). Growth failure is a problem in children with congenital heart disease (CHD), most of all in children with heart failure due to left-to-right shunts (Daymont et al., 2013b). In South India, Vaidyanathan and colleagues (Vaidyanathan et al., 2006) reported a high prevalence of underweight (59%) and wasting (55,9%) in children with CHD. This group reported that growth failure is not always reversed by corrective interventions. In developing countries, because of resource limitations, corrective interventions for CHD are performed late, leading to a vicious cycle of congestive heart failure and respiratory infections (Kumar & Shrivastava, 2008). It is important to identify the aetiology of poor growth in CHD to guide attempts to improve growth and mental development (Ravishankar et al., 2013). The beta-blocker propranolol effectively reduces stress in infants with heart failure due to congenital heart disease which is indicated by an improvement of heart rate variability in 24 hour Holter ECG's (Buchhorn et al., 2002a). Together with R. Motz (Motz et al., 2005) we found a highly significant positive correlation between weight gain and the vagal parameters rMSSD ($p<0.01$) and pNN50 ($p<0.001$) in infants with congenital heart disease and these parameters improve after propranolol therapy.

For a better understanding of the programming effect of heart failure in infancy we intend to perform a follow up examination in patients of the VSD-PHF trial initiated by the All Indian Institute of Medical where since 2008 infants with VSD received propranolol or standard therapy for heart failure in a prospective, randomized trial.

Meanwhile the effect of beta-blockade on autonomic maturation is demonstrated in a neonate with severe heart failure caused by myocarditis. One day after the switch from dobutamine to carvedilol the neonate showed a dramatic increase of total power and decrease of NT-Pro-BNP levels.

Taken together, malnutrition in utero and ex utero (Manhardt et al., 2010) or early life stress due to congenital heart disease (Paul et al., 2009) have an effect on HRV and NT-Pro-BNP levels independent from heart disease. In later life these patients have a higher risk for cognitive disorders like ADHD (Heinonen et al., 2010;Boyle et al., 2011;Ramel & Georgieff, 2014) and a higher cardiovascular risk. We speculate a programming effect of early life stress on the autonomous nervous system indicated by a lifelong reduced

HRV. Stress prevention during the "first 1000 days of life" by optimal care and nutrition of mothers and child may prevent later cardiovascular and/or mental disease. If "stress" is not preventable, most of all in infants with severe disease like heart failure, patients need a pharmacological blockade by beta-blockers that may possibly prevent a lifelong autonomic regulation disorder.

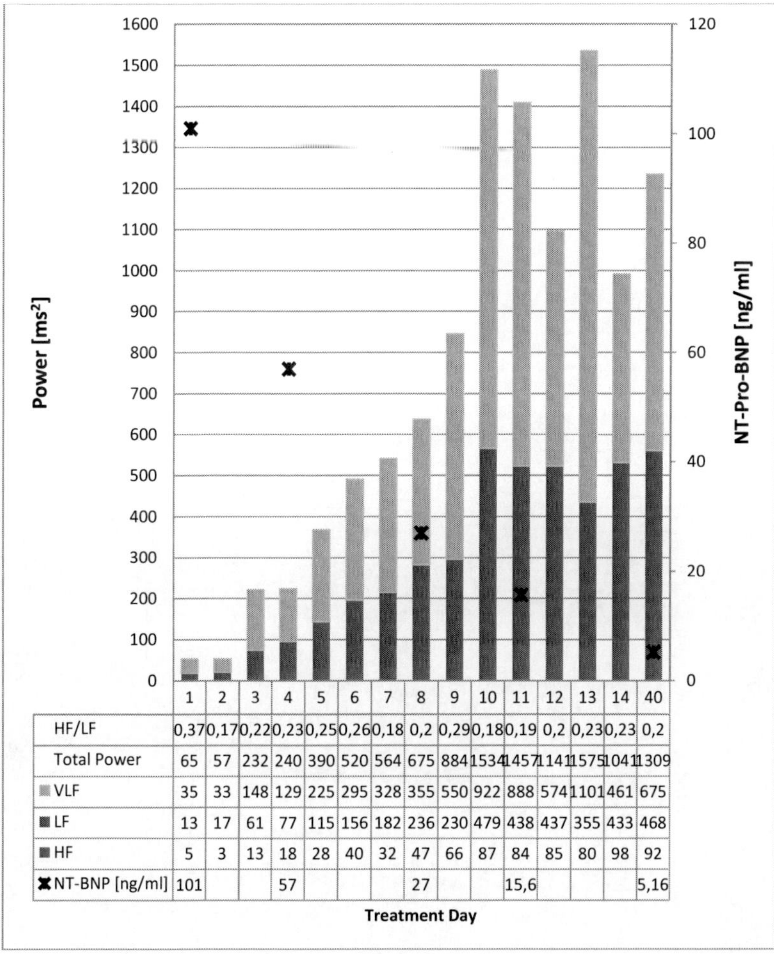


| | 1 | 2 | 3 | 4 | 5 | 6 | 7 | 8 | 9 | 10 | 11 | 12 | 13 | 14 | 40 |
|---|---|---|---|---|---|---|---|---|---|---|---|---|---|---|---|
| HF/LF | 0,37 | 0,17 | 0,22 | 0,23 | 0,25 | 0,26 | 0,18 | 0,2 | 0,29 | 0,18 | 0,19 | 0,2 | 0,23 | 0,23 | 0,2 |
| Total Power | 65 | 57 | 232 | 240 | 390 | 520 | 564 | 675 | 884 | 1534 | 1457 | 1141 | 1575 | 1041 | 1309 |
| VLF | 35 | 33 | 148 | 129 | 225 | 295 | 328 | 355 | 550 | 922 | 888 | 574 | 1101 | 461 | 675 |
| LF | 13 | 17 | 61 | 77 | 115 | 156 | 182 | 236 | 230 | 479 | 438 | 437 | 355 | 433 | 468 |
| HF | 5 | 3 | 13 | 18 | 28 | 40 | 32 | 47 | 66 | 87 | 84 | 85 | 80 | 98 | 92 |
| NT-BNP [ng/ml] | 101 | | | 57 | | | | 27 | | | 15,6 | | | | 5,16 |

Treatment Day

Figure 9.3. Effect of the switch from dobutamine to carvedilol therapy at day 3 on HRV and NT-Pro-BNP in a neonate with severe heart failure due to myocarditis.

*Chapter 10*

# HRV and Death

"If the pattern of the heart beat becomes as regular as the tapping of a wood-pecker or the dripping of rain from the roof, the patient will be dead in 4 days." This sentence is the most often citation of the Chinese physician Wang Su Ho (265—317 A.D) to show that HRV predict prognosis. A huge number of publications underline the prognostic value of HRV analysis in nearly all disease and age groups (Dekker et al., 1997). But perhaps there are even more specific HRV patterns beneath the statistical analysis of HRV parameters for prediction of sudden cardiac death.

For further explanation some case studies from children who died or have had to be resuscitated without cardiovascular disease are demonstrated. This has been possible by an online HRV monitoring system in our intensive care unit that uses routine monitor data. The first case is a five year old boy with near sudden unexpected death in epilepsy (SUDEP). He had to be resuscitated in our intensive care unit after prolonged generalized tonic-clonic seizures. The etiology of his seizures and severe mental retardation remains unclear but MR imaging shows progressive brain atrophy that begun in early infancy. He stayed in hospital to change his antiepileptic drug therapy because of an increasing number of daily generalized tonic-clonic seizures. After prolonged generalized tonic-clonic seizures during intensive care monitoring he developed severe hypopnea and had to be intubated but showed no signs of circulatory failure or heart rhythm disturbances. At this time he was treated with 120 mg/kg/d valproic acid, 10 mg/kg/d vigabatrin, 2,5 mg/kg/d phenobarbital, 5 mg/kg/d topiramat and 10 μg/kg/d clonidine. Intoxication was excluded by drug monitoring (valproic acid: 51.5 μg/ml; Phenobarbital: 20.5 μg/ml; topiramat: 9.1 mg/l clonidine:<0.1 μg/l). The boy developed severe lung failure but he was weaned from respirator after one week without additional neurological problems. Because we were aware of the high risk of sudden unexpected death from epilepsy and the crucial role of autonomic dysfunction in this child we used 24hours Holter ECG monitoring for risk stratification over a time period of more than 6 years. The results of a total number of 14 Holter ECG's are illustrated in the Figure 10.1. The most impressive changes concerned parasympathetic activity expressed as rMSSD values. Compared to 5 Holter ECG's within one year before near SUDEP, the Holter ECG's during the hospital stay when near SUDEP occurred showed an impressive reduction of HRV and a complete loss of circadian rhythm indicated by a high HRV Score. We treated the boy with 3mg/kg L-Dopa beside antiepileptic drug therapy of valproic acid and phenobarbital. The Holter ECG monitoring showed an impressive increase of parasympathetic activity during nightime over 4 years (Figure 10.2). Under this therapy he never developed further life threatening hypopnoea.

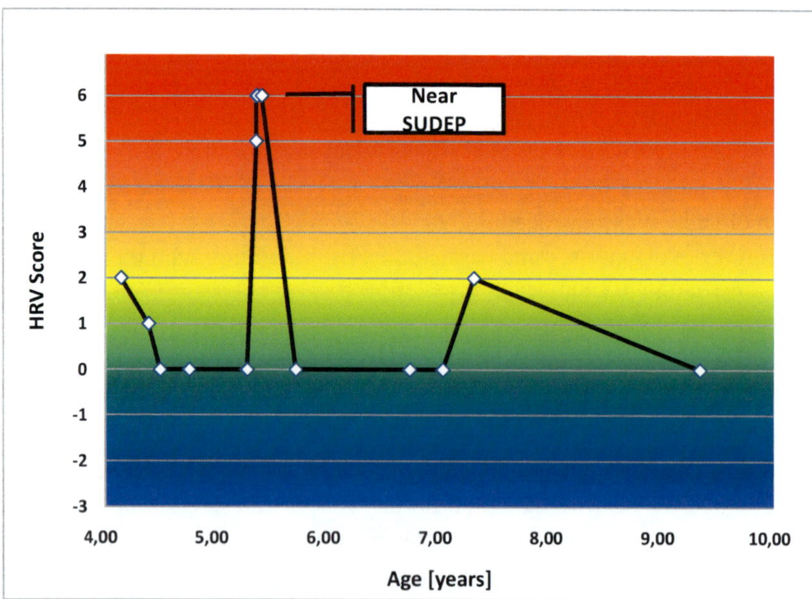


Figure 10.1. 6 year HRV Monitoring in a boy with refractory generalized epilepsy who had to be resuscitated during hospital stay to change antiepileptic drug therapy at the age of 5.5 years (Near SUDEP).

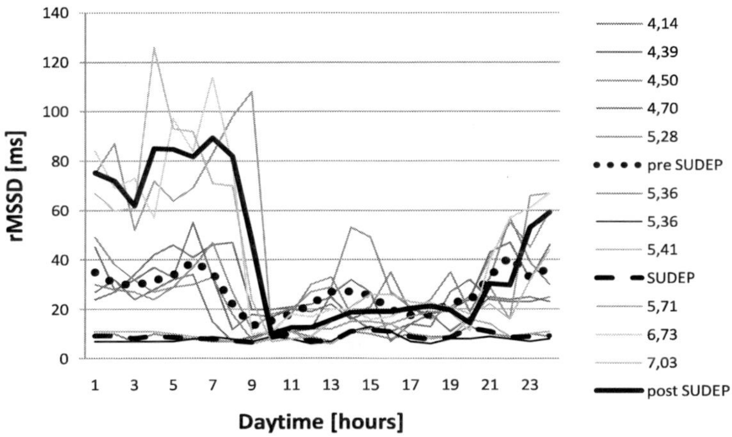


Figure 10.2. Circadian parasympathetic activity in eleven 24 hours Holter ECG's expressed as hourly rMSSD values [ms] of a boy with a history of generalized tonic-clonic seizures and severe mental retardation between the of the age of 4 and 9 years. The bold lines describe the average values of five Holter ECG's before near SUDEP (pre SUDEP), three Holter ECG's immediately at the time of near SUDEP (SUDEP) and three Holter ECG's after near SUDEP (post SUDEP).

Sudden unexpected death in epilepsy is the most common cause of death directly related to epilepsy and tends to occur in young people with refractory epilepsy because HRV in children with refractory epilepsy is significantly lower than normal (Raju et al., 2012), the increased sympathetic tone in association with decreased parasympathetic tone may constitute the mechanism underlying sudden unexpected death in epilepsy (DeGiorgio et al., 2010). In this case, HRV analysis on the day before near SUDEP and in other cases on the day before death showed unusual heart rate patterns (regular short decelerations) and/or very uniform waves in Fast Fourier Analysis (Figure 10.3). After a successful resuscitation these patterns disappeared as shown in case 4. Given that case 5 has a zero line encephalogram these unusual uniform patterns of the Fast Fourier powerplot which are most clearly indicated in case 3 and 5, could be a resonance pattern generated in the brainstem. Only these two cases received a palliative treatment without catecholamines and other drugs or procedures that may have interfered with the dying process. I am convinced that dying is an active process and medical treatment may be helpful or harmful. A better understanding of the dying process is an important indicator of good clinical practice. Perhaps Wang Su Ho and the "Medicus" in the popular film could feel this pulse phenomenon and their "premonition of death" was an important part of their legendary reputation.

Case 1: Day before near SUDEP

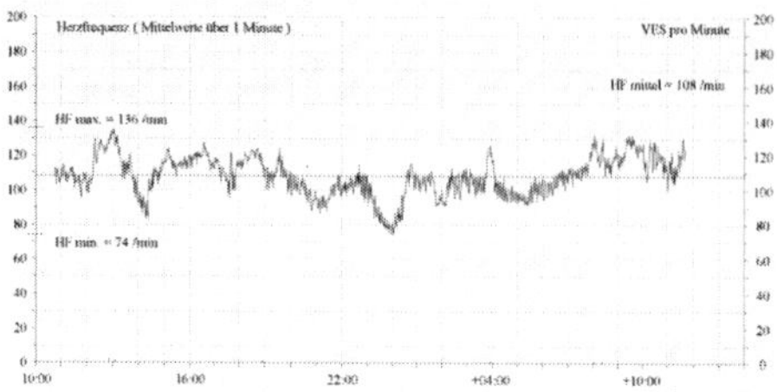


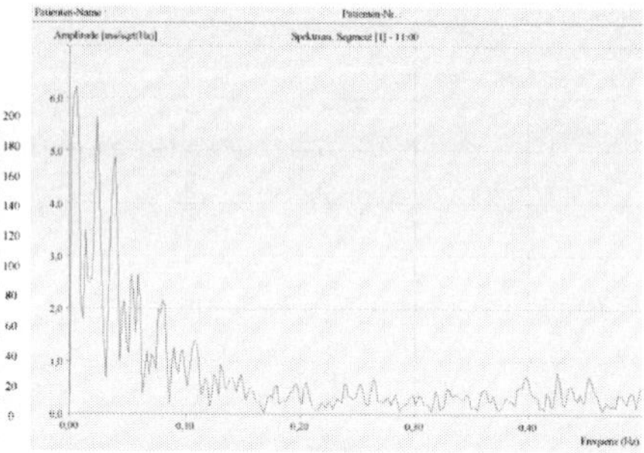


Case 2: Day before death due to chronic lung failure

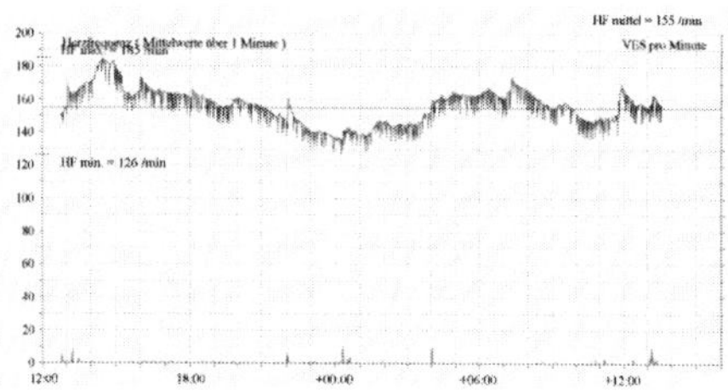


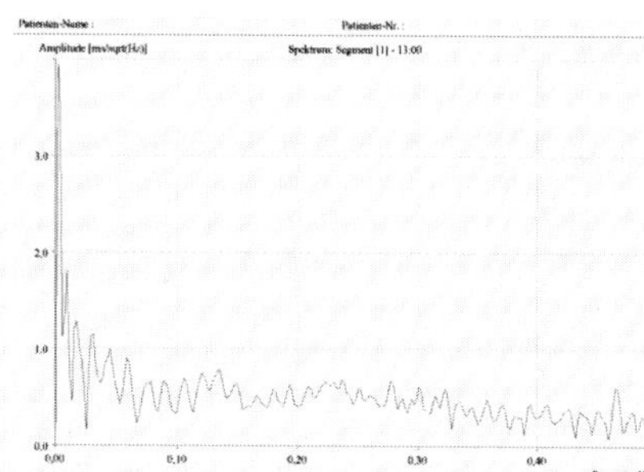


Case 3: Day before death due to a brain tumor

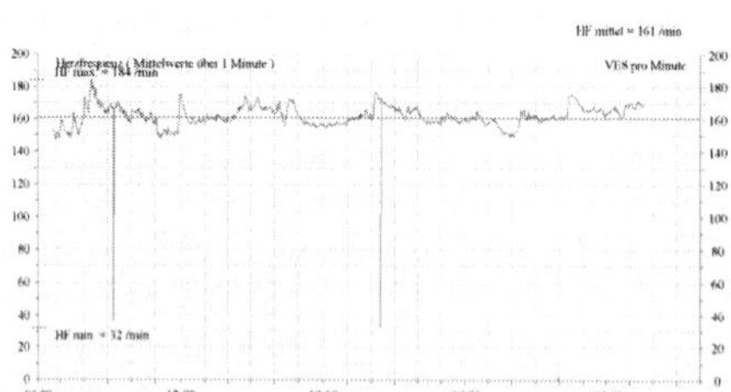


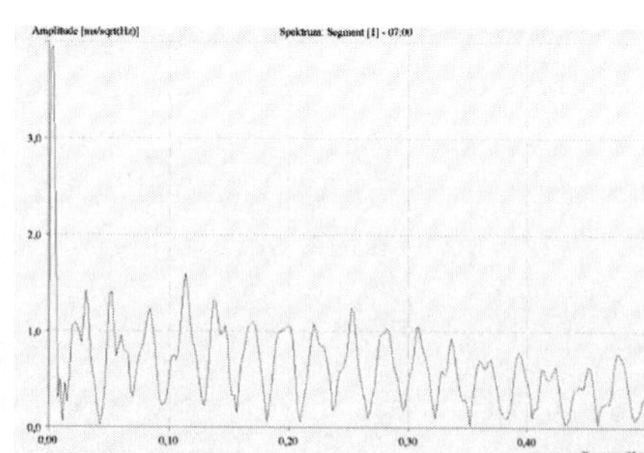

Case 4a: Day before resuscitation due to lung failure

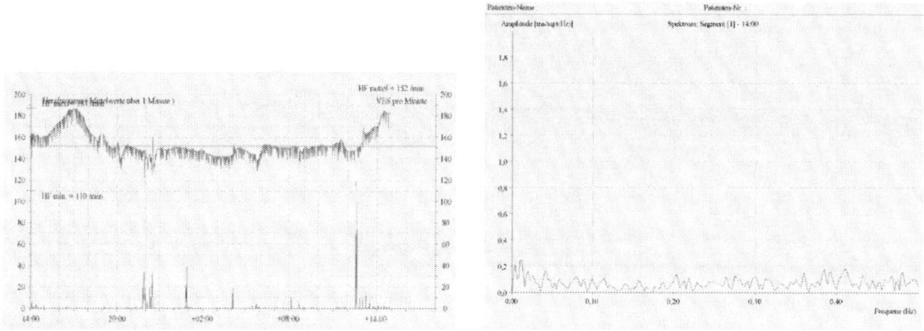

Case 4b: Same patient at the last day of hospital stay

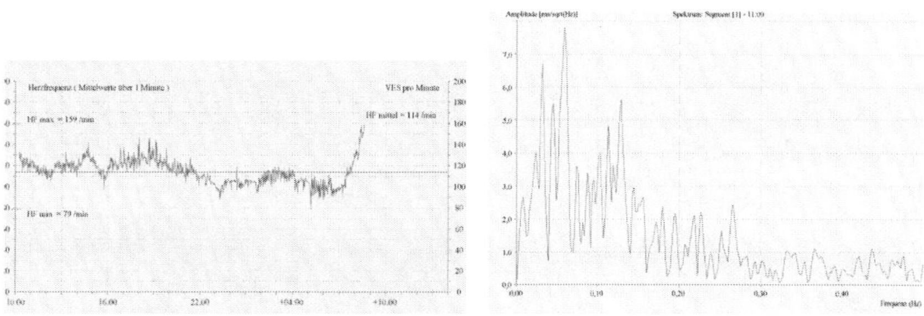

Case 5: 5 day old newborn after perinatal asphyxia, brain death

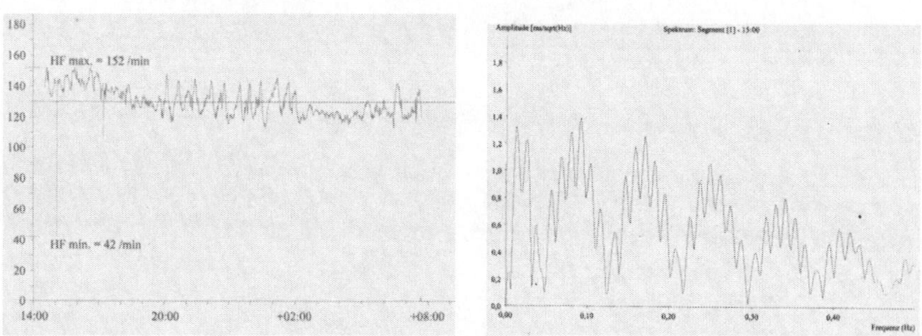


Figure 10.3. HRV analysis in children at the day before death or resuscitation.

# Conclusion

Based upon the hypothesis that prognosis in childhood heart failure depends on autonomic dysfunction, I introduced a new heart failure model and a medical therapy with beta-blockers in 1996. We used the analysis of heart rate variability (HRV) in 24 hours Holter ECG's for the understanding of the pathophysiology of childhood heart failure and for objective control of medical therapy. HRV in infants with congenital heart disease prior to surgery is related to heart failure and significantly improved during propranolol therapy but not during a standard medical therapy with digoxin and diuretics.

Clinical studies in childhood heart failure are lacking and this new methodological approach was necessary for proper therapeutic decisions based on evidence-based clinical concept. Together with other pioneers of beta-blocker therapy in childhood heart failure, we have recently been able to demonstrate in a review article the long-term beneficial effects of this new clinical approach (Buchhorn & Ross, 2014b).

The success of this clinical model was the inspiration of a new approach to mental disease in childhood. In the last decades, an increase of new paediatric problems requiring medical care like eating disorders, behavioural and attention problems has been observed. This so called "New Morbidities in Childhood" is accompanied by increasing costs for mental health and cardiovascular disease in all age groups. All these diseases are related to autonomic dysfunction and have a high impact on cardiovascular prognosis. Based upon the hypothesis that behavioural problems are accompanied by changes in the autonomic nervous system, we have performed analysis of HRV in 24 hours Holter ECG's since 2005. Measurements taken between an age of 1 to 40 years have been collected in the following groups: healthy children with respect to school affiliation; a historical control group from literature published in 1997; attention deficit disorder with and without hyperactivity; anorexia nervosa and obesity. This data was compared to children with an increased cardiovascular risk due to congenital heart disease. In order to analyse the effect of autonomic function on human growth, we measured HRV in children with growth failure. A new HRV Score was established for the comparison of autonomic function in different age groups.

We could demonstrate a decrease of vagal activity in healthy children of today and speculate that insufficient vagal maturation may be a reason for an increasing prevalence of mental and cardiovascular disease. Looking for the reason of this vagal shift caloric over nutrition, omega-3-fatty acid deficiency, high intensity of information and communication technology usage and some environmental toxins reduce HRV in childhood.

HRV is related to body mass index with low HRV in obesity and high HRV in children with anorexia nervosa. Based upon our data we could demonstrate an association of caloric intake with autonomic function in children using HRV analysis. Growth failure in children with growth hormone deficiency and small for gestational age but not in children with constitutional growth delay is related to autonomic dysfunction. Children with attention deficit- and somatoform disorders had significantly reduced vagal activity that was more reduced than those of children with congenital heart disease. We further speculate that fetal/neonatal autonomic programming by caloric under or over nutrition in- and/or ex utero or heart failure in infants is a cause of a lifelong autonomic dysfunction with the well-known consequences of an enhanced cardiovascular risk, cognitive disorders, obesity and/or stunting in these patients.

The effect of methylphenidate, growth hormone therapy, clonidine and beta-blockers on autonomic function in children are discussed.

# References

(1996). Heart rate variability: standards of measurement, physiological interpretation and clinical use. Task Force of the European Society of Cardiology and the North American Society of Pacing and Electrophysiology. *Circulation* 93, 1043-1065.

Acevedo, M., Corbalan, R., Chamorro, G., Jalil, J., Nazzal, C., Campusano, C., & Castro, P. (2003). Administration of growth hormone to patients with advanced cardiac heart failure: effects upon left ventricular function, exercise capacity, and neurohormonal status. *Int.J.Cardiol.* 87, 185-191.

Akcaboy, M., Atalay, S., Ucar, T., & Tutar, E. (2011). Heart rate variability during asymptomatic periods in children with recurrent neurocardiogenic syncope. *Turk.J.Pediatr.* 53, 59-66.

Amichai, T. & Katz-Leurer, M. (2014). Heart rate variability in children with cerebral palsy: review of the literature and meta-analysis. *NeuroRehabilitation.* 35, 113-122.

Aulakh, C. S., Hill, J. L., & Murphy, D. L. (1994). Attenuation of clonidine-induced growth hormone release following chronic glucocorticoid and 5-hydroxytryptamine uptake-inhibiting antidepressant treatments. *Neuroendocrinology* 59, 35-41.

Ayton, A. K., Azaz, A., & Horrobin, D. F. (2004). A pilot open case series of ethyl-EPA supplementation in the treatment of anorexia nervosa. *Prostaglandins Leukot.Essent.Fatty Acids* 71, 205-209.

Aziz, W., Schlindwein, F. S., Wailoo, M., Biala, T., & Rocha, F. C. (2012). Heart rate variability analysis of normal and growth restricted children. *Clin.Auton.Res.* 22, 91-97.

Bae, S., Kim, J. H., Lim, Y. H., Park, H. Y., & Hong, Y. C. (2012). Associations of bisphenol A exposure with heart rate variability and blood pressure. *Hypertension* 60, 786-793.

Barutcu, I., Esen, A. M., Kaya, D., Turkmen, M., Karakaya, O., Saglam, M., Melek, M., Celik, A., Kilit, C., Onrat, E., & Kirma, C. (2011). Do mobile phones pose a potential risk to autonomic modulation of the heart? *Pacing Clin.Electrophysiol.* 34, 1511-1514.

Battipaglia, I., Scalone, G., Macchione, A., Pinnacchio, G., Laurito, M., Milo, M., Pelargonio, G., Bencardino, G., Bellocci, F., Pieroni, M., Lanza, G. A., & Crea, F. (2012). Association of heart rate variability with arrhythmic events in patients with arrhythmogenic right ventricular cardiomyopathy/dysplasia. *Circ.J.* 76, 618-623.

Baum, P., Petroff, D., Classen, J., Kiess, W., & Bluher, S. (2013). Dysfunction of autonomic nervous system in childhood obesity: a cross-sectional study. *PLoS.One.* 8, e54546.

Ben Dov, I. Z., Kark, J. D., Ben Ishay, D., Mekler, J., Ben Arie, L., & Bursztyn, M. (2007). Blunted heart rate dip during sleep and all-cause mortality. *Arch.Intern.Med.* 167, 2116-2121.

Billman, G. E. (2012). Omega-3 polyunsaturated fatty acids and cardiac rhythm: an introduction. *Front Physiol* 3, 457.

Billman, G. E. (2013a). The effect of heart rate on the heart rate variability response to autonomic interventions. *Front Physiol* 4, 222.

Billman, G. E. (2013b). The effects of omega-3 polyunsaturated fatty acids on cardiac rhythm: a critical reassessment. *Pharmacol.Ther.* 140, 53-80.

Billman, G. E. (2013c). The LF/HF ratio does not accurately measure cardiac sympatho-vagal balance. *Front Physiol* 4, 26.

Birch, S. L., Duncan, M. J., & Franklin, C. (2012). Overweight and reduced heart rate variability in British children: an exploratory study. *Prev.Med.* 55, 430-432.

Bomba, M., Corbetta, F., Gambera, A., Nicosia, F., Bonini, L., Neri, F., Tremolizzo, L., & Nacinovich, R. (2014). Heart rate variability in adolescents with functional hypothalamic amenorrhea and anorexia nervosa. *Psychiatry Res.* 215, 406-409.

Boneva, R. S., Decker, M. J., Maloney, E. M., Lin, J. M., Jones, J. F., Helgason, H. G., Heim, C. M., Rye, D. B., & Reeves, W. C. (2007). Higher heart rate and reduced heart rate variability persist during sleep in chronic fatigue syndrome: a population-based study. *Auton.Neurosci.* 137, 94-101.

Bonnemeier, H., Richardt, G., Potratz, J., Wiegand, U. K., Brandes, A., Kluge, N., & Katus, H. A. (2003a). Circadian profile of cardiac autonomic nervous modulation in healthy subjects: differing effects of aging and gender on heart rate variability. *J.Cardiovasc.Electrophysiol.* 14, 791-799.

Boyle, M. H., Miskovic, V., Van Lieshout, R., Duncan, L., Schmidt, L. A., Hoult, L., Paneth, N., & Saigal, S. (2011). Psychopathology in young adults born at extremely low birth weight. *Psychol.Med.* 41, 1763-1774.

Buchhorn, R. & Christian, W. (2013a). Ventricular arrhythmias in children with attention deficit disorder - a symptom of autonomic imbalance? *Cardiol.Young.* 1-6.

Buchhorn, R., Conzelmann, A., Willaschek, C., Stork, D., Taurines, R., & Renner, T. J. (2012a). Heart rate variability and methylphenidate in children with ADHD. *Atten.Defic.Hyperact.Disord.* 4, 85-91.

Buchhorn, R., Hammersen, A., Bartmus, D., & Bursch, J. (2001a). The pathogenesis of heart failure in infants with congenital heart disease. *Cardiol.Young.* 11, 498-504.

Buchhorn, R., Hulpke-Wette, M., Hilgers, R., Bartmus, D., Wessel, A., & Bursch, J. (2001b). Propranolol treatment of congestive heart failure in infants with congenital heart disease: The CHF-PRO-INFANT Trial. Congestive heart failure in infants treated with propanol. *Int.J.Cardiol.* 79, 167-173.

Buchhorn, R., Hulpke-Wette, M., Nothroff, J., & Paul, T. (2002a). Heart rate variability in infants with heart failure due to congenital heart disease: reversal of depressed heart rate variability by propranolol. *Med.Sci.Monit.* 8, CR661-CR666.

Buchhorn, R. & McConnell, M. E. (2014). Beta blockers in childhood heart failure - why not? *Int.J.Cardiol.* 175, 211-212.

Buchhorn, R., Muller, C., Willaschek, C., & Norozi, K. (2012b). How to predict the impact of methylphenidate on cardiovascular risk in children with attention deficit disorder: methylphenidate improves autonomic dysfunction in children with ADHD. *ISRN.Pharmacol.* 2012, 170935.

Buchhorn, R. & Ross, R. D. (2014a). The Long Way to a Successful Medical Therapy of Heart Failure with Beta-blockers in Children with Heart Disease. *Rev.Recent Clin.Trials.*

Buchhorn, R., Ross, R. D., Bartmus, D., Wessel, A., Hulpke-Wette, M., & Bursch, J. (2001c). Activity of the renin-angiotensin-aldosterone and sympathetic nervous system and their relation to hemodynamic and clinical abnormalities in infants with left-to-right shunts. *Int.J.Cardiol.* 78, 225-230.

Buchhorn, R., Ziemer, G., Jetter, H. M., Borst, M., & Selbach, J. (2014). Renal sympathetic denervation for resistant hypertension in a child after aortic coarctation surgery. *Int.J.Cardiol.* 172, e447-e448.

Butera, G., Bonnet, D., Iserin, L., Sidi, D., Kachaner, J., & Villain, E. (1999). Total cavopulmonary and atriopulmonary connections are associated with reduced heart rate variability. *Heart* 82, 704-707.

Capalbo, D., Raso, G. M., Esposito, A., Mase, R. D., Barbieri, F., Meli, R., Bruzzese, D., & Salerno, M. (2013). Cluster Of Cardiometabolic Risk Factors In Children With Gh Deficiency: A Prospective, Case-Control Study. *Clin.Endocrinol.(Oxf).*

Carel, J. C., Ecosse, E., Landier, F., Meguellati-Hakkas, D., Kaguelidou, F., Rey, G., & Coste, J. (2012). Long-term mortality after recombinant growth hormone treatment for isolated growth hormone deficiency or childhood short stature: preliminary report of the French SAGhE study. *J.Clin.Endocrinol.Metab* 97, 416-425.

Cooper, W. O., Habel, L. A., Sox, C. M., Chan, K. A., Arbogast, P. G., Cheetham, T. C., Murray, K. T., Quinn, V. P., Stein, C. M., Callahan, S. T., Fireman, B. H., Fish, F. A., Kirshner, H. S., O'Duffy, A., Connell, F. A., & Ray, W. A. (2011a). ADHD drugs and serious cardiovascular events in children and young adults. *N.Engl.J.Med.* 365, 1896-1904.

da Silva, C. C., Pereira, L. M., Cardoso, J. R., Moore, J. P., & Nakamura, F. Y. (2014). The effect of physical training on heart rate variability in healthy children: a systematic review with meta-analysis. *Pediatr.Exerc.Sci.* 26, 147-158.

Dalsgaard, S., Kvist, A. P., Leckman, J. F., Nielsen, H. S., & Simonsen, M. (2014). Cardiovascular safety of stimulants in children with attention-deficit/hyperactivity disorder: a nationwide prospective cohort study. *J.Child Adolesc.Psychopharmacol.* 24, 302-310.

Davos, C. H., Davlouros, P. A., Wensel, R., Francis, D., Davies, L. C., Kilner, P. J., Coats, A. J., Piepoli, M., & Gatzoulis, M. A. (2002a). Global impairment of cardiac autonomic nervous activity late after repair of tetralogy of Fallot. *Circulation* 106, I69-I75.

Daymont, C., Neal, A., Prosnitz, A., & Cohen, M. S. (2013a). Growth in children with congenital heart disease. *Pediatrics* 131, e236-e242.

De Bock, F., Jarczok, M. N., Hoffmann, K., & Buchhorn, R. (2013). Do our children lose vagus activity? Potential time trends of children's autonomic nervous system activity. *Int.J.Cardiol.* 170, e30-e32.

DeGiorgio, C. M., Miller, P., Meymandi, S., Chin, A., Epps, J., Gordon, S., Gornbein, J., & Harper, R. M. (2010). RMSSD, a measure of vagus-mediated heart rate variability, is associated with risk factors for SUDEP: the SUDEP-7 Inventory. *Epilepsy Behav.* 19, 78-81.

Dekker, J. M., Schouten, E. G., Klootwijk, P., Pool, J., Swenne, C. A., & Kromhout, D. (1997). Heart rate variability from short electrocardiographic recordings predicts mortality from all causes in middle-aged and elderly men. The Zutphen Study. *Am.J.Epidemiol.* 145, 899-908.

Diamond, A. (2012). Executive Functions. *Annu.Rev.Psychol.*

Dippacher, S., Willaschek, C., & Buchhorn, R. (2014). Different nutritional states and autonomic imbalance in childhood. *Eur.J.Clin.Nutr.*

Doksoz, O., Oner, T., Guven, B., Karaarslan, U., Ozdemir, R., Yozgat, Y., Mese, T., Tavli, V., Okur, F. F., & Alayunt, E. A. (2014). Mid-term assessment of cardiac autonomic functions in children with transposition of the great arteries after arterial switch operation. *Anadolu.Kardiyol. Derg.*

Fan, X., Hua, W., Xu, Y., Ding, L., Niu, H., Chen, K., Xu, B., & Zhang, S. (2014). Incidence and predictors of sudden cardiac death in patients with reduced left ventricular ejection fraction after myocardial infarction in an era of revascularisation. *Heart* 100, 1242-1249.

Fei, L., Anderson, M. H., Katritsis, D., Sneddon, J., Statters, D. J., Malik, M., & Camm, A. J. (1994). Decreased heart rate variability in survivors of sudden cardiac death not associated with coronary artery disease. *Br.Heart J.* 71, 16-21.

Florant, G. L. & Healy, J. E. (2012). The regulation of food intake in mammalian hibernators: a review. *J.Comp Physiol B* 182, 451-467.

Folino, A. F., Russo, G., Bauce, B., Mazzotti, E., & Daliento, L. (2004). Autonomic profile and arrhythmic risk stratification after surgical repair of tetralogy of Fallot. *Am.Heart J.* 148, 985-989.

Garcia-Ortiz, L., Garcia-Garcia, A., Ramos-Delgado, E., Patino-Alonso, M. C., Recio-Rodriguez, J. I., Rodriguez-Sanchez, E., & Gomez-Marcos, M. A. (2011). Relationships of night/day heart rate ratio with carotid intima media thickness and markers of arterial stiffness. *Atherosclerosis* 217, 420-426.

Giagkoudaki, F., Dimitros, E., Kouidi, E., & Deligiannis, A. (2010). Effects of exercise training on heart-rate-variability indices in individuals with Down Syndrome. *J.Sport Rehabil.* 19, 173-183.

Glazier, D. S. (2014). Is metabolic rate a universal 'pacemaker' for biological processes? *Biol.Rev.Camb.Philos.Soc.*

Gutin, B., Howe, C., Johnson, M. H., Humphries, M. C., Snieder, H., & Barbeau, P. (2005). Heart rate variability in adolescents: relations to physical activity, fitness, and adiposity. *Med.Sci.Sports Exerc.* 37, 1856-1863.

Habel, L. A., Cooper, W. O., Sox, C. M., Chan, K. A., Fireman, B. H., Arbogast, P. G., Cheetham, T. C., Quinn, V. P., Dublin, S., Boudreau, D. M., Andrade, S. E., Pawloski, P. A., Raebel, M. A., Smith, D. H., Achacoso, N., Uratsu, C., Go, A. S., Sidney, S., Nguyen-Huynh, M. N., Ray, W. A., & Selby, J. V. (2011). ADHD medications and risk of serious cardiovascular events in young and middle-aged adults. *JAMA* 306, 2673-2683.

Hastings, M., O'Neill, J. S., & Maywood, E. S. (2007). Circadian clocks: regulators of endocrine and metabolic rhythms. *J.Endocrinol.* 195, 187-198.

Heinonen, K., Raikkonen, K., Pesonen, A. K., Andersson, S., Kajantie, E., Eriksson, J. G., Wolke, D., & Lano, A. (2010). Behavioural symptoms of attention deficit/hyperactivity disorder in preterm and term children born small and appropriate for gestational age: a longitudinal study. *BMC.Pediatr.* 10, 91.

Henje, B. E., Olsson, E. M., Serlachius, E., Ericson, M., & Ingvar, M. (2009). Heart rate variability is related to self-reported physical activity in a healthy adolescent population. *Eur.J.Appl.Physiol* 106, 877-883.

Hill, K. D., Chiswell, K., Califf, R. M., Pearson, G., & Li, J. S. (2014). Characteristics of pediatric cardiovascular clinical trials registered on ClinicalTrials.gov. *Am.Heart J.* 167, 921-929.

Jaiswal, M., Urbina, E. M., Wadwa, R. P., Talton, J. W., D'Agostino, R. B., Jr., Hamman, R. F., Fingerlin, T. E., Daniels, S., Marcovina, S. M., Dolan, L. M., & Dabelea, D. (2013). Reduced heart rate variability among youth with type 1 diabetes: the SEARCH CVD study. *Diabetes Care* 36, 157-162.

Janes, R. D., Brandys, J. C., Hopkins, D. A., Johnstone, D. E., Murphy, D. A., & Armour, J. A. (1986). Anatomy of human extrinsic cardiac nerves and ganglia. *Am.J.Cardiol.* 57, 299-309.

Jelinek, H. F., Md, I. H., Al Aubaidy, H., & Khandoker, A. H. (2013). Association of cardiovascular risk using non-linear heart rate variability measures with the framingham risk score in a rural population. *Front Physiol* 4, 186.

Judges, D., Beverly, S., Rio, A., & Goff, L. M. (2012). Clinical guidelines and enteral nutrition support: a survey of dietetic practice in the United Kingdom. *Eur.J.Clin.Nutr.* 66, 130-135.

Kaur, G., Phillips, C., Wong, K., & Saini, B. (2013). Timing is important in medication administration: a timely review of chronotherapy research. *Int.J.Clin.Pharm.*

Kumar, R. K. & Shrivastava, S. (2008). Paediatric heart care in India. *Heart* 94, 984-990.

Lachish, M., Stein, D., Kaplan, Z., Matar, M., Faigin, M., Korsunski, I., & Cohen, H. (2009). Irreversibility of cardiac autonomic dysfunction in female adolescents diagnosed with anorexia nervosa after short- and long-term weight gain. *World J.Biol.Psychiatry* 10, 503-511.

Lacour-Gayet, F. & Clarke, D. R. (2005). The Aristotle method: a new concept to evaluate quality of care based on complexity. *Curr.Opin.Pediatr.* 17, 412-417.

Leong, K. S., Mann, P., Wallymahmed, M., MacFarlane, I. A., & Wilding, J. P. (2000). Abnormal heart rate variability in adults with growth hormone deficiency. *J.Clin.Endocrinol.Metab* 85, 628-633.

Leong, K. S., Mann, P., Wallymahmed, M., MacFarlane, I. A., & Wilding, J. P. (2001). The influence of growth hormone replacement on heart rate variability in adults with growth hormone deficiency. *Clin.Endocrinol.(Oxf)* 54, 819-826.

Lin, P. C., Kuo, S. Y., Lee, P. H., Sheen, T. C., & Chen, S. R. (2014). Effects of internet addiction on heart rate variability in school-aged children. *J.Cardiovasc.Nurs.* 29, 493-498.

Lo, S. C., Ravaldi, C., Cabras, P. L., Faravelli, C., & Ricca, V. (2008). Stress, hypothalamic-pituitary-adrenal axis and eating disorders. *Neuropsychobiology* 57, 95-115.

Lotufo, P. A., Valiengo, L., Bensenor, I. M., & Brunoni, A. R. (2012). A systematic review and meta-analysis of heart rate variability in epilepsy and antiepileptic drugs. *Epilepsia* 53, 272-282.

Lou, Y., Peng, W. J., Cao, Y., Cao, D. S., Xie, J., & Li, H. H. (2014). The effectiveness of propranolol in treating infantile haemangiomas: a meta-analysis including 35 studies. *Br.J.Clin.Pharmacol.* 78, 44-57.

Ma, Q. L., Wang, B., Fu, G. H., Chen, G. F., & Chen, Z. Y. (2011). [Heart rate variability in children with beta-thalassemia major]. *Zhongguo Dang.Dai Er.Ke.Za Zhi.* 13, 654-656.

Manhardt, L. B., Norozi, K., Muller, C., Willaschek, C., Kostuch, B., & Buchhorn, R. (2010). NT-Pro-B-Type Natriuretic Peptide Levels in Infants with Failure to Thrive due to Caloric Deprivation. *Int.J.Pediatr.* 2010, 983468.

Massin, M. & von Bernuth, G. (1997). Normal ranges of heart rate variability during infancy and childhood. *Pediatr.Cardiol.* 18, 297-302.

McElhinney, D. B., Colan, S. D., Moran, A. M., Wypij, D., Lin, M., Majzoub, J. A., Crawford, E. C., Bartlett, J. M., McGrath, E. A., & Newburger, J. W. (2004). Recombinant human growth hormone treatment for dilated cardiomyopathy in children. *Pediatrics* 114, e452-e458.

McLennan, P. L. (2014). Cardiac physiology and clinical efficacy of dietary fish oil clarified through cellular mechanisms of omega-3 polyunsaturated fatty acids. *Eur.J.Appl.Physiol* 114, 1333-1356.

Michels, N., Clays, E., De Buyzere, M., Vanaelst, B., De Henauw, S., & Sioen, I. (2013). Children's sleep and autonomic function: low sleep quality has an impact on heart rate variability. *Sleep* 36, 1939-1946.

Moisiadis, V. G. & Matthews, S. G. (2014). Glucocorticoids and fetal programming part 2: Mechanisms. *Nat.Rev.Endocrinol.* 10, 403-411.

Montgomery, P., Burton, J. R., Sewell, R. P., Spreckelsen, T. F., & Richardson, A. J. (2014). Fatty acids and sleep in UK children: subjective and pilot objective sleep results from the DOLAB study--a randomized controlled trial. *J.Sleep Res.* 23, 364-388.

Mortensen, S. A., Rosenfeldt, F., Kumar, A., Dolliner, P., Filipiak, K. J., Pella, D., Alehagen, U., Steurer, G., & Littarru, G. P. (2014). The Effect of Coenzyme Q on Morbidity and Mortality in Chronic Heart Failure: Results From Q-SYMBIO: A Randomized Double-Blind Trial. *JACC.Heart Fail.*

Motz, R., Harding, P., Quick, P., Kramer, H. H., Allgeier, B., & Buchhorn, R. (2005). Is heart rate variability an objective parameter with which to manage treatment of infants with heart failure due to left-to-right shunting? *Cardiol.Young.* 15, 8-12.

Mrosovsky, N. & Powley, T. L. (1977). Set points for body weight and fat. *Behav.Biol.* 20, 205-223.

Nissen, S. E. (2006). ADHD drugs and cardiovascular risk. *N.Engl.J.Med.* 354, 1445-1448.

Norozi, K., Bahlmann, J., Raab, B., Alpers, V., Arnhold, J. O., Kuehne, T., Klimes, K., Zoege, M., Geyer, S., Wessel, A., & Buchhorn, R. (2007). A prospective, randomized, double-blind, placebo controlled trial of beta-blockade in patients who have undergone surgical correction of tetralogy of Fallot. *Cardiol.Young.* 17, 372-379.

Nyberg, C. H., Leonard, W. R., Tanner, S., McDade, T., Huanca, T., & Godoy, R. A. (2012a). Diurnal cortisol rhythms and child growth:

exploring the life history consequences of HPA activation among the Tsimane'. *Am.J.Hum.Biol.* 24, 730-738.

Oflaz, M. B., Balli, S., Kibar, A. E., Ece, I., Akdeniz, C., & Tuzcu, V. (2013). Effects of carvedilol therapy on cardiac autonomic control, QT dispersion, and ventricular arrhythmias in children with dilated cardiomyopathy. *Med.Sci.Monit.* 19, 366-372.

Ohuchi, H., Negishi, J., Miyake, A., Sakaguchi, H., Miyazaki, A., & Yamada, O. (2011). Long-term prognostic value of cardiac autonomic nervous activity in postoperative patients with congenital heart disease. *Int.J.Cardiol.* 151, 296-302.

Ohuchi, H., Takasugi, H., Ohashi, H., Yamada, O., Watanabe, K., Yagihara, T., & Echigo, S. (2004). Abnormalities of neurohormonal and cardiac autonomic nervous activities relate poorly to functional status in fontan patients. *Circulation* 110, 2601-2608.

Ononogbu, S., Wallenius, M., Punamaki, R. L., Saarni, L., Lindholm, H., & Nygard, C. H. (2014). Association between Information and Communication Technology Usage and the Quality of Sleep among School-Aged Children during a School Week. *Sleep Disord.* 2014, 315808.

Paajanen, T. A., Oksala, N. K., Kuukasjarvi, P., & Karhunen, P. J. (2010). Short stature is associated with coronary heart disease: a systematic review of the literature and a meta-analysis. *Eur.Heart J.* 31, 1802-1809.

Pal, G. K., Chandrasekaran, A., Hariharan, A. P., Dutta, T. K., Pal, P., Nanda, N., & Venugopal, L. (2012a). Body mass index contributes to sympathovagal imbalance in prehypertensives. *BMC.Cardiovasc.Disord.* 12, 54.

Pal, G. K., Pal, P., Nanda, N., Lalitha, V., Dutta, T. K., & Adithan, C. (2012c). Sympathovagal Imbalance in Young Prehypertensives: Importance of Male-Female Difference. *Am.J.Med.Sci.*

Park, S. K., Auchincloss, A. H., O'Neill, M. S., Prineas, R., Correa, J. C., Keeler, J., Barr, R. G., Kaufman, J. D., & Diez Roux, A. V. (2010). Particulate air pollution, metabolic syndrome, and heart rate variability: the multi-ethnic study of atherosclerosis (MESA). *Environ.Health Perspect.* 118, 1406-1411.

Paul, M. A., Backer, C. L., Binns, H. J., Mavroudis, C., Webb, C. L., Yogev, R., & Franklin, W. H. (2009). B-Type Natriuretic Peptide and Heart Failure in Patients with Ventricular Septal Defect: A Pilot Study. *Pediatr.Cardiol.*

Petretta, M., Bonaduce, D., Scalfi, L., De Filippo, E., Marciano, F., Migaux, M. L., Themistoclakis, S., Ianniciello, A., & Contaldo, F. (1997). Heart rate variability as a measure of autonomic nervous system function in anorexia nervosa. *Clin.Cardiol.* 20, 219-224.

Petryk, A., Baker, K. S., Frohnert, B., Moran, A., Chow, L., Sinaiko, A. R., Steffen, L. M., Perkins, J. L., Zhang, L., Hodges, J. S., & Steinberger, J. (2013). Blunted response to a growth hormone stimulation test is associated with unfavorable cardiovascular risk factor profile in childhood cancer survivors. *Pediatr.Blood Cancer* 60, 467-473.

Pieters, N., Plusquin, M., Cox, B., Kicinski, M., Vangronsveld, J., & Nawrot, T. S. (2012). An epidemiological appraisal of the association between heart rate variability and particulate air pollution: a meta-analysis. *Heart* 98, 1127-1135.

Porges, S. W. (2009). The polyvagal theory: new insights into adaptive reactions of the autonomic nervous system. *Cleve.Clin.J.Med.* 76 Suppl 2, S86-S90.

Raju, K. N., Choudhary, N., Gulati, S., Kabra, M., Jaryal, A. K., Deepak, K. K., & Pandey, R. M. (2012). Comparison of heart rate variability among children with well controlled versus refractory epilepsy: a cross-sectional study. *Epilepsy Res.* 101, 88-91.

Ramel, S. E. & Georgieff, M. K. (2014). Preterm nutrition and the brain. *World Rev.Nutr.Diet.* 110, 190-200.

Ravishankar, C., Zak, V., Williams, I. A., Bellinger, D. C., Gaynor, J. W., Ghanayem, N. S., Krawczeski, C. D., Licht, D. J., Mahony, L., Newburger, J. W., Pemberton, V. L., Williams, R. V., Sananes, R., Cook, A. L., Atz, T., Khaikin, S., & Hsu, D. T. (2013). Association of impaired linear growth and worse neurodevelopmental outcome in infants with single ventricle physiology: a report from the pediatric heart network infant single ventricle trial. *J.Pediatr.* 162, 250-256.

Reynolds, R. M., Labad, J., Buss, C., Ghaemmaghami, P., & Raikkonen, K. (2013). Transmitting biological effects of stress in utero: implications for mother and offspring. *Psychoneuroendocrinology* 38, 1843-1849.

Reynolds, R. M., Walker, B. R., Syddall, H. E., Andrew, R., Wood, P. J., Whorwood, C. B., & Phillips, D. I. (2001). Altered control of cortisol secretion in adult men with low birth weight and cardiovascular risk factors. *J.Clin.Endocrinol.Metab* 86, 245-250.

Richardson, T., Rozkovec, A., Thomas, P., Ryder, J., Meckes, C., & Kerr, D. (2004). Influence of caffeine on heart rate variability in patients with long-standing type 1 diabetes. *Diabetes Care* 27, 1127-1131.

Risnes, K. R., Vatten, L. J., Baker, J. L., Jameson, K., Sovio, U., Kajantie, E., Osler, M., Morley, R., Jokela, M., Painter, R. C., Sundh, V., Jacobsen, G. W., Eriksson, J. G., Sorensen, T. I., & Bracken, M. B. (2011). Birthweight and mortality in adulthood: a systematic review and meta-analysis. *Int.J.Epidemiol.* 40, 647-661.

Rocks, T., Pelly, F., & Wilkinson, P. (2014). Nutrition therapy during initiation of refeeding in underweight children and adolescent inpatients with anorexia nervosa: a systematic review of the evidence. *J.Acad.Nutr.Diet.* 114, 897-907.

Scolnick, B., Mostofsky, D. I., & Keane, R. J. (2014). Pilot study employing heart rate variability biofeedback training to decrease anxiety in patients with eating disorders. *J.Eat.Disord.* 2, 17.

Silvetti, M. S., Drago, F., & Ragonese, P. (2001). Heart rate variability in healthy children and adolescents is partially related to age and gender. *Int.J.Cardiol.* 81, 169-174.

Simeone, P. & Alberti, S. (2014). Epigenetic heredity of human height. *Physiol Rep.* 2.

Sokolovic, N., Kuriyan, R., Kurpad, A. V., & Thomas, T. (2013). Sleep and birthweight predict visceral adiposity in overweight/obese children. *Pediatr.Obes.*

Spencer, S. J. (2013). Perinatal programming of neuroendocrine mechanisms connecting feeding behavior and stress. *Front Neurosci.* 7, 109.

Stapelberg, N. J., Hamilton-Craig, I., Neumann, D. L., Shum, D. H., & McConnell, H. (2012). Mind and heart: heart rate variability in major depressive disorder and coronary heart disease - a review and recommendations. *Aust.N.Z.J.Psychiatry* 46, 946-957.

Staud, R. (2008). Heart rate variability as a biomarker of fibromyalgia syndrome. *Fut.Rheumatol.* 3, 475-483.

Tanriverdi, F., Eryol, N. K., Atmaca, H., Unluhizarci, K., Ozdogru, I., Sarikaya, I., Bayram, F., & Kelestimur, F. (2005). The effects of 12 months of growth hormone replacement therapy on cardiac autonomic tone in adults with growth hormone deficiency. *Clin.Endocrinol.(Oxf)* 62, 706-712.

Tascilar, E., Yokusoglu, M., Dundaroz, R., Baysan, O., Ozturk, S., Yozgat, Y., & Kilic, A. (2009). Cardiac autonomic imbalance in children with allergic rhinitis. *Tohoku J.Exp.Med.* 219, 187-191.

Thayer, J. F., Ahs, F., Fredrikson, M., Sollers, J. J., III, & Wager, T. D. (2012). A meta-analysis of heart rate variability and neuroimaging studies:

implications for heart rate variability as a marker of stress and health. *Neurosci.Biobehav.Rev.* 36, 747-756.

Thayer, J. F. & Lane, R. D. (2007). The role of vagal function in the risk for cardiovascular disease and mortality. *Biol.Psychol.* 74, 224-242.

Thayer, J. F. & Lane, R. D. (2009). Claude Bernard and the heart-brain connection: further elaboration of a model of neurovisceral integration. *Neurosci.Biobehav.Rev.* 33, 81-88.

Thayer, J. F., Yamamoto, S. S., & Brosschot, J. F. (2010a). The relationship of autonomic imbalance, heart rate variability and cardiovascular disease risk factors. *Int.J.Cardiol.* 141, 122-131.

Tong, H., Rappold, A. G., Diaz-Sanchez, D., Steck, S. E., Berntsen, J., Cascio, W. E., Devlin, R. B., & Samet, J. M. (2012). Omega-3 fatty acid supplementation appears to attenuate particulate air pollution-induced cardiac effects and lipid changes in healthy middle-aged adults. *Environ.Health Perspect.* 120, 952-957.

Umetani, K., Singer, D. H., McCraty, R., & Atkinson, M. (1998). Twenty-four hour time domain heart rate variability and heart rate: relations to age and gender over nine decades. *J.Am.Coll.Cardiol.* 31, 593-601.

Unalacak, M., Aydin, M., Ermis, B., Ozeren, A., Sogut, A., Demirel, F., & Unluoglu, I. (2004). Assessment of cardiac autonomic regulation in children with monosymptomatic nocturnal enuresis by analysis of heart rate variability. *Tohoku J.Exp.Med.* 204, 63-69.

Vaidyanathan, B., Roth, S. J., Gauvreau, K., Shivaprakasha, K., Rao, S. G., & Kumar, R. K. (2006). Somatic growth after ventricular septal defect in malnourished infants. *J.Pediatr.* 149, 205-209.

Valera, B., Muckle, G., Poirier, P., Jacobson, S. W., Jacobson, J. L., & Dewailly, E. (2012). Cardiac autonomic activity and blood pressure among Inuit children exposed to mercury. *Neurotoxicology* 33, 1067-1074.

Vaseghi, M. & Shivkumar, K. (2008). The role of the autonomic nervous system in sudden cardiac death. *Prog.Cardiovasc.Dis.* 50, 404-419.

Vincenti, A., Brambilla, R., Fumagalli, M. G., Merola, R., & Pedretti, S. (2006). Onset mechanism of paroxysmal atrial fibrillation detected by ambulatory Holter monitoring. *Europace.* 8, 204-210.

Wabitsch, M., Kunze, D., Keller, E., Kiess, W., & Kromeyer-Hauschild, K. (2002). [Ever more children and adolescents are overweight. How can the obesity epidemic be stopped?]. *MMW.Fortschr.Med.* 144, 30-34.

Weber, C. S., Thayer, J. F., Rudat, M., Wirtz, P. H., Zimmermann-Viehoff, F., Thomas, A., Perschel, F. H., Arck, P. C., & Deter, H. C. (2010). Low vagal tone is associated with impaired post stress recovery of cardiovascular, endocrine, and immune markers. *Eur.J.Appl.Physiol* 109, 201-211.

Weiss, E. P. & Fontana, L. (2011). Caloric restriction: powerful protection for the aging heart and vasculature. *Am.J.Physiol Heart Circ.Physiol* 301, H1205-H1219.

Weitz, G., Bonnemeier, H., Sufke, S., Wellhoner, P., Lehnert, H., & Dodt, C. (2013). Heart rate variability and metabolic rate in healthy young adults with low birth weight. *Am.J.Cardiovasc.Dis.* 3, 239-246.

Wenstrom, K. D. (2014). The FDA's new advice on fish: it's complicated. *Am.J.Obstet.Gynecol.*

Widenhorn-Muller, K., Schwanda, S., Scholz, E., Spitzer, M., & Bode, H. (2014). Effect of supplementation with long-chain omega-3 polyunsaturated fatty acids on behavior and cognition in children with attention deficit/hyperactivity disorder (ADHD): a randomized placebo-controlled intervention trial. *Prostaglandins Leukot.Essent.Fatty Acids* 91, 49-60.

Wu, L., Jiang, Z., Li, C., & Shu, M. (2014). Prediction of heart rate variability on cardiac sudden death in heart failure patients: A systematic review. *Int.J.Cardiol.* 174, 857-860.

Zhang, J., Fang, S. C., Mittleman, M. A., Christiani, D. C., & Cavallari, J. M. (2013). Secondhand tobacco smoke exposure and heart rate variability and inflammation among non-smoking construction workers: a repeated measures study. *Environ.Health* 12, 83.

Zhou, Y., Xie, G., Wang, J., & Yang, S. (2012). Cardiovascular risk factors significantly correlate with autonomic nervous system activity in children. *Can.J.Cardiol.* 28, 477-482.

Zulfiqar, U., Jurivich, D. A., Gao, W., & Singer, D. H. (2010a). Relation of high heart rate variability to healthy longevity. *Am.J.Cardiol.* 105, 1181-1185.

# Index


## $\alpha_2$

$\alpha_2$-adrenoceptor, 77, 78, 82, 93, 94
$\alpha_2$-adrenoreceptor subsensitivity, 78, 82

## A

abdominal pain, 49
abuse, 39
accelerated idioventricular rhythm, 65
access, 55
acetylation, 94
acid, 36, 40, 41, 42, 43, 45, 62, 99, 106, 118
AD, 45, 46, 47
ADHD, ix, 3, 5, 13, 17, 40, 45, 46, 47, 65, 66, 89, 90, 91, 96, 109, 110, 112, 114, 119
adiposity, 112
adolescents, 2, 3, 4, 5, 13, 22, 32, 48, 87, 93, 108, 112, 113, 117, 118
adrenoceptors, 77, 78, 82
adulthood, 24, 68, 117
adults, 5, 6, 9, 15, 18, 40, 48, 55, 56, 64, 65, 69, 73, 76, 77, 82, 83, 89, 91, 112, 113, 117, 118
aetiology, 96
age, 3, 5, 7, 8, 11, 13, 17, 24, 27, 42, 43, 45, 46, 49, 58, 60, 63, 64, 71, 73, 76, 79, 80, 81, 82, 83, 84, 99, 100, 101, 105, 117, 118
agonist, 77
aldosterone, 56, 109
allergic rhinitis, 117
ambient air, 43, 115
amenorrhea, 32, 108
amines, 65, 89
angiotensin converting enzyme, 63
anorexia, 21, 24, 26, 32, 33, 34, 35, 36, 37, 38, 39, 93, 106, 107, 108, 113, 116, 117
anorexia nervosa, 21, 24, 32, 34, 37, 93, 106, 107, 108, 116, 117
ANOVA, 21
antibiotic, 62
antidepressant, 107
antiepileptic drug therapy, 99, 100
antiepileptic drugs, 113
anxiety, 117
aorta, 58
aortic coarctation, 71, 110
aortic valve, 62
Aristotle, 58, 59, 113
arithmetic, ix, 1
arrhythmia(s), 1, 4, 17, 40, 41, 45, 65, 66, 69, 70, 87, 109, 115
arrhythmogenic right ventricular dysplasia, 66
arterial hypertension, 17, 27, 71
arteries, 58, 111

artery, 58
assessment, 65, 111
asthma, 55
asymptomatic, 86, 107
atherosclerosis, 43, 111, 115
athletes, 11
atrial fibrillation, 69, 118
atrophy, 99
Attention Deficit Hyperactivity Disorder, ix, 4
autonomic activity, 118
autonomic nervous system, vii, viii, 1, 11, 15, 17, 24, 25, 26, 27, 49, 55, 58, 64, 65, 68, 69, 93, 105, 108, 110, 116, 118, 119
autonomic programming, 58, 89, 106
autonomic switch, 34, 36, 82

## B

base, 82
BB-BUCH trial, 86
beneficial effect, 40, 84, 86, 105
benefits, 40, 51, 84
beta-blocker(s), vii, 18, 32, 34, 49, 62, 63, 83, 84, 85, 87, 88, 96, 97, 105, 106, 109
biofeedback, 18, 36, 117
biofeedback training, 36, 117
biological processes, 26, 111
biomarker, 58, 117
birth weight, 18, 26, 73, 109, 116, 119
births, 14
birthweight, 76, 117
Bisoprolol, 86
bisphenol, 108
Bisphenol A (BPA), ix, 43
blood, 17, 45, 71, 108, 118
blood pressure, 17, 45, 71, 89, 108, 118
BMI, ix, 23, 28, 29, 30, 32, 34, 35, 36, 43, 46, 48, 62, 75
body mass index, 17, 18, 21, 28, 36, 37, 46, 62, 71, 106
body weight, 35, 36, 114
bradycardia, 38
brain, 2, 15, 66, 86, 99, 116, 118
brainstem, 101
breast feeding, 93, 94
breathing, 26
Britain, 17

## C

caffeine, 18, 91, 117
7caloric intake, 18, 26, 27, 31, 34, 106
caloric reduction, 32
caloric restriction, 34
candidates, 73
cardiac arrest, 65
cardiac arrhythmia, 1, 45
cardiac autonomic function, 111
cardiac risk, 65
cardiac surgery, 57, 58, 59, 84
cardiomyopathies, 63, 87
cardiomyopathy, 3, 63, 64, 66, 67, 83, 108, 114, 115
cardiovascular disease, 13, 15, 55, 73, 99, 105, 106, 118
cardiovascular morbidity, 14
cardiovascular mortality, 82
cardiovascular risk, 18, 27, 31, 43, 64, 65, 73, 77, 78, 82, 93, 96, 106, 109, 112, 114, 116
Cardiovascular Risk, 17
cardiovascular side effects, 65
carvedilol, 63, 64, 83, 87, 96, 97, 115
case studies, 99
case study, 35
catecholamines, 101
central nervous system, 27
cerebral palsy, 49, 107
chemical, 43
CHF, 84, 109
childhood, vii, 5, 8, 13, 15, 17, 21, 26, 28, 29, 30, 31, 42, 43, 48, 55, 77, 82, 105, 106, 108, 109, 110, 111, 114, 116
childhood cancer, 77, 116
China, 17
chronic fatigue, 41, 48, 49, 108
chronic fatigue syndrome, 41, 48, 49, 108
chronopharmacotherapy, 32
chronotherapy, 113

circadian rhythm(s), 5, 26, 27, 65, 100
classes, 4
clinical symptoms, 56
clinical trials, 55, 112
clonidine, 18, 77, 78, 79, 80, 81, 82, 99, 106, 107
coarctation, 71, 110
coenzyme, 63
cognition, 119
color, 4, 10
communication, ix, 19, 43, 106
competition, viii
complexity, 58, 59, 113
complications, 66
composition, 26
conduct disorder, 13
congenital heart defects, 49, 56, 60, 61, 68
congenital heart disease(s), 49, 55, 58, 59, 61, 84, 86, 96, 105, 106, 109, 110, 115
congenital malformations, 55
congestive heart failure, 96, 109
construction, 119
consumption, 14, 42, 43, 51, 52, 53
control group, 5, 15, 24, 47, 80, 81, 89, 105
controlled trials, 51
coronary artery disease, 64, 111
coronary heart disease, 115, 117
correlation, 7, 15, 24, 26, 58, 65
correlations, 63
cortisol, 78, 115, 116
cost, 13
cross-sectional study, 21, 27, 108, 116
CVD, 112
cyanotic, 58
cycling, 5

## D

data analysis, 1
defects, 49, 56, 57, 58, 60, 61, 68, 82, 87
deficiency, 73, 74, 77, 78, 79, 80, 81, 83, 93, 106, 110, 113, 117
deficit, vii, 3, 13, 17, 21, 39, 41, 65, 89, 106, 109, 110, 112, 119
demographic change, 14
Denmark, 91
depression, 14, 15
desensitization, 18
developing countries, 96
deviation, x, 1, 10
diabetes, viii, 84
Diabetes mellitus, 51
Digoxin, 62, 84, 86
dilated cardiomyopathy, 3, 83, 114, 115
diseases, vii, 11, 14, 16, 17, 39, 55, 73, 78, 105
disorder, vii, 3, 13, 17, 18, 21, 39, 41, 48, 56, 65, 89, 97, 106, 109, 110, 112, 119
dispersion, 115
distribution, 15
Diuretics, 84, 86
DNA, 94
dobutamine, 96, 97
doctors, viii
dominance, 17, 28, 32, 34, 36, 71, 73, 82
dose-response relationship, 91
Down syndrome, 51
drug therapy, 69, 99, 100
drugs, 40, 55, 101, 110, 114
Duchenne, 63, 64, 67
dysplasia, 66, 108

## E

Early life stress, 93
eating disorders, 13, 105, 113, 117
education, 28
EEG, 2
elaboration, 118
electrocardiogram, 65
electromagnetic, 15, 43
electromagnetic fields, 43
electromagnetic waves, 15
e-mail, viii
emotional disorder, 15, 18
endocarditis, 62
endocrine, 51, 112, 119
energy, 26
energy expenditure, 26
enteric nervous system, 26

enuresis, 118
environmental tobacco, 43
environmental toxins, 19, 43, 106
EPA, 107
epidemic, 14, 118
epigenetic, 93, 94
epilepsy, 49, 99, 100, 101, 113, 116
equipment, 7, 9
etiology, 99
Europe, 55, 82
evidence, 18, 26, 31, 40, 43, 56, 65, 68, 84, 89, 93, 94, 105, 117
examinations, 2
executive function, 27
executive functions, 27
exercise, 5, 51, 65, 107, 111
exertion, 51
exposure, 42, 43, 94, 108, 119
eye movement, 18

## F

failure to thrive, 56, 93
Fallot, 62, 63, 86, 87, 110, 111, 114
Fast Fourier Analysis, ix, 2, 28, 31, 35, 40, 42, 101
fat, 114
fatigue syndrome, 40, 41, 48, 49, 108
fatty acids, 18, 32, 34, 40, 42, 49, 65, 68
FDA, 42, 119
fetus, 94
fibromyalgia, 40, 48, 49, 117
financial, viii
financial support, viii
Fire of Life, 4, 39
first 1000 days of life, 97
fish, 40, 42, 62, 114, 119
fish oil, 40, 114
fitness, 112
flight, 27
fluctuations, 26
food, 26, 43, 111
Food and Drug Administration, 89
food intake, 26, 111
formula, 94
France, 17
Frequency Domain Analysis, 2, 7
frontal cortex, 27
funds, 18

## G

gene expression, 94
generalized tonic-clonic seizure, 99, 101
genetics, 15
Germany, vii, viii, 4, 5, 13, 14, 16, 17, 71
gestational age, 73, 74, 78, 79, 80, 81, 93, 106, 112
globalization, 14
glucocorticoid(s), 94, 107
glucose, 32
glucose tolerance, 32
good clinical practice, 101
Great Britain, 17
growth, vii, viii, 18, 73, 74, 75, 76, 77, 78, 79, 80, 81, 82, 83, 84, 93, 96, 106, 107, 110, 113, 114, 115, 116, 117, 118
growth hormone, 18, 73, 74, 75, 77, 78, 79, 80, 81, 82, 83, 84, 93, 106, 107, 110, 113, 114, 116, 117
growth hormone stimulation test, 77, 78, 116
guidelines, 113

## H

haemangiomatosis, 88
headache, 48, 87
health, 13, 82, 118
healthy control patient, 3, 38, 45
heart disease, vii, 49, 55, 56, 58, 59, 61, 63, 65, 73, 74, 83, 84, 86, 88, 96, 105, 106, 109, 110, 115, 117
heart failure, vii, 3, 5, 17, 27, 49, 55, 56, 57, 58, 63, 64, 66, 67, 82, 83, 84, 85, 86, 87, 88, 93, 96, 97, 105, 106, 107, 109, 114, 119
Heart rate:, 1
heart transplantation, 83

height, 73, 77, 82, 89, 93, 117
hepatomegaly, 56
heredity, 117
hibernating circuit, 34
hibernation, 26
high blood pressure, 89
high school, 46, 47, 52
histone, 94
historical data, 36
history, 48, 65, 78, 101, 115
hormone, 73, 74, 75, 77, 78, 82, 83, 84, 106, 110, 113, 117
hospitalization, 35
HPA axis, 26, 27
HRV monitoring, 63
HRV Score, 8, 9, 10, 11, 56, 57, 58, 59, 60, 61, 62, 63, 64, 67, 68, 71, 74, 100, 106
human, vii, 5, 77, 93, 106, 112, 114, 117
hydrocortisone, 78
hyperactivity, 3, 106, 110, 112, 119
hypertension, 17, 27, 31, 32, 43, 71, 110
hypothalamic regulation, 32
hypothalamus, 2, 26, 27, 93
hypothesis, vii, 15, 18, 27, 51, 56, 105

## I

ideal, 3, 15, 26
idiopathic, 78
imbalances, 73
immunadsorption therapy, 63
immune markers, 52, 119
in utero, 96, 116
incidence, 15, 17, 18, 46, 65, 66
India, 17, 71, 96, 113
individuals, 73, 111
infancy, 10, 24, 49, 58, 82, 89, 93, 96, 99, 114
infants, vii, 49, 55, 56, 57, 58, 64, 82, 84, 86, 93, 94, 96, 97, 105, 106, 109, 114, 116, 118
infection, 15
infectious mononucleosis, 48
inflammation, 119
inhibition, 78, 84
inhibitor, 77
initial state, 38
initiation, 37, 82, 117
injury, 48
institutions, vii
integration, 18, 118
intensive care unit, 99
intervention, 18, 32, 37, 119
intima, 111
intrauterine growth retardation, 73
intrinsic pacemaker rate, 26, 27, 28, 34, 40
ischemic heart disease, 73
issues, 27
Italy, 17

## K

kidney, 71

## L

later life, 15, 96
lead, 94
learning, 38, 46, 47
learning difficulties, 46, 47
left to right shunt, 55
left ventricular dysfunction, 63
lesions, 84
leukemia, 55
life style, 62, 63
lifetime, 6, 15
limbic system, 2, 27
lipid metabolism, 32
longevity, 119
longitudinal study, 78, 112
low birthweight, 76
lying, 6, 24

## M

magnetic resonance, 2
magnetic resonance imaging, 2
major depression, 13, 18
major depressive disorder, 117

majority, 31
malnutrition, 49, 96
management, 84
mass, 21, 26, 31, 71, 115
maternal stress, 94
matter, 43
measurement(s), viii, 7, 34, 43, 45, 65, 107
media, 14, 18, 43, 51, 52, 53, 111
medical, vii, 47, 48, 55, 62, 63, 65, 83, 101, 105
medical care, 105
medication, 18, 113
mellitus, viii, 51, 84
memory, 34
mental development, 93, 96
mental disorder, 13, 48, 82, 93
mental health, 13, 18, 105
mental retardation, 99, 101
mercury, 42, 118
Mercury, 42
meta-analysis, 107, 110, 113, 115, 116, 117, 118
metabolic rate, 26, 27, 111, 119
metabolic syndrome, viii, 32, 43, 115
metabolism, 26
metabolized, 90
methylation, 94
methylphenidate, ix, 3, 13, 14, 18, 45, 46, 65, 89, 90, 91, 106, 109
metoprolol, 65
microRNA, 94
misunderstanding, 89
mobile phone, 43, 108
models, 26, 94
mononucleosis, 48
mood disorder, 13
morbidity, 13, 73
morphology, 56
mortality, vii, 14, 32, 55, 64, 73, 82, 84, 108, 110, 111, 117, 118
MR, 99
MRI, ix, 2
multi-ethnic, 115
myocardial infarction, 64, 111
myocarditis, 63, 96, 97

## N

nasogastric tube, 36
natriuretic peptides, 58
negative emotions, 34
neonates, 58
nephron, 83, 84
nerve, 57
nerve fibers, 57
nervous system, 15, 18, 26, 34, 55, 58, 64, 71, 90, 96
neurocognitive disorders, 94
neurohormonal, 56, 83, 107, 115
Neurohormonal inhibition, 84
neuroimaging, 118
neurological disease, 77
NICE protocol, 35, 36, 37
norepinephrine, 56, 58, 84, 96
normal distribution, 15
North America, 107
NT-Pro-BNP, 58, 59, 63, 93, 96, 97
nuclei, 26, 27
nutrient, 26
nutrition, viii, 14, 17, 18, 21, 34, 36, 37, 94, 97, 106, 113, 116
nutritional state, 22, 23, 24, 25, 32, 111

## O

obesity, vii, 13, 21, 23, 27, 28, 29, 30, 31, 46, 51, 62, 106, 108, 118
obstruction, 84
omega 3 fatty acids, 18, 32, 40, 42, 49, 65
omega-3, 34, 42, 45, 62, 68, 106, 108, 114, 119
online HRV monitoring, 99
outpatient, 77
overweight, 21, 24, 28, 117, 118
oxygen, 58, 61, 62, 86

## P

pacemaker rate, 27, 40
pain, vii, 48

palliative, 58, 60, 101
parasympathetic activity, 27, 100, 101
parasympathetic nervous system, 1, 26
parents, 13
paroxysmal atrial fibrillation, 69, 118
paroxysmal supraventricular tachycardia, 68, 69, 70
paroxysmal tachycardia, 69
particulate air pollution, 43, 116, 118
pathogenesis, 109
Pathophysiologic Model, 14
pathophysiological, 27, 46, 64, 66, 77
pathophysiology, 105
pathways, 78
peptide(s), 58, 86
percentile, 21, 23, 29, 77, 82
peristalsis, 15
phthalates, 19
physical activity, 18, 51, 52, 112
physical training, 28, 51, 110
physiology, 114, 116
pilot study, 89
placebo, 114, 119
PM, ix
pollution, 19, 43, 115, 116, 118
polyunsaturated fat, 108, 114, 119
polyunsaturated fatty acids, 108, 114, 119
polyvagal theory, 15, 27, 116
population, 2, 65, 108, 112
positive correlation, 96
posttraumatic stress, 18
premature ventricular contractions, 65, 66, 68
prematurity, 49
prevention, 58, 97
proarrhythmogenic effects, 65, 89
proband(s), 3, 52
professionals, viii
prognosis, vii, 14, 71, 99, 105
prognostic value, 3, 99, 115
programming, 18, 58, 78, 89, 93, 94, 95, 96, 106, 114, 117
project, vii, 82
propranolol, 58, 88, 96, 105, 109, 113
protection, 43, 119
psychiatric disorders, 13, 14, 18, 66
psychiatry, 14
psychosocial stress, 78
psychosomatic, 11, 78
puberty, 15
public health, 13
PVC, ix, 67, 87

## Q

quality of life, 63

## R

reactions, 116
recognition, vii, 14
recommendations, 65, 117
recovery, 5, 51, 52, 53, 119
re-feeding, 32, 33, 34, 35, 36, 37, 38, 39, 94
regression, 5, 16, 24, 89
regression line, 24
rehabilitation, 34
relaxation, 18
relevance, 84
renal failure, 83, 84
renal sympathetic denervation, 71
renin, 56, 84, 109
repair, 110, 111
reprocessing, 18
reputation, 101
requirements, 5
resection, 71
resistance, 34
respirator, 100
response, 26, 27, 77, 108, 116
retardation, 78
Reynolds Medical Systems, 7
rhythm, 26, 47, 65, 89, 99, 108
right atrium, 58
risk, 6, 17, 31, 32, 45, 52, 62, 64, 65, 68, 73, 77, 82, 89, 91, 93, 94, 96, 100, 108, 111, 112, 118, 119
risk factors, 62, 111, 118, 119

rMSSD, ix, 1, 5, 7, 9, 10, 15, 17, 23, 24, 27, 28, 29, 34, 35, 38, 41, 43, 45, 46, 47, 48, 49, 51, 64, 65, 66, 69, 70, 73, 74, 75, 78, 79, 80, 86, 87, 88, 89, 96, 100, 101
Road Map, 18
root, ix, 1
Ross Score, 56, 57, 84, 86, 87
rural population, 112

## S

safety, 110
Schiller Company, 7
school, 4, 42, 46, 47, 48, 93, 105, 113
school performance, 93
school success, 46, 48
SDNN, x, 1, 5, 9, 10, 15, 17, 21, 23, 24, 25, 27, 28, 29, 34, 35, 41, 43, 46, 48, 49, 56, 62, 69, 73, 74, 75, 82, 86, 87, 88
secretion, 77, 78, 116
sensitivity, 56
sexual abuse, 39
short time HRV, 26
showing, 3, 13, 24
side effects, 65, 89
signs, 56, 84, 99
Singapore, 17
sinus arrhythmia, 4
sinus rhythm, 1
sleep, 22, 26, 43, 45, 69, 108, 114
sleep disturbance, 45
small for gestational age, 73, 106
small gestational age, 74, 78, 79, 80, 81, 93
smoking, 62, 119
sNN50/pNN50, 1
society, 14, 78
somatoform disorder(s), 40, 45, 48, 49, 106
spiroergometry, 58, 62
sports, 17, 51, 52, 53, 62
standard deviation, 9, 24, 46, 73, 74, 75
Standard values, 5
starvation, 38, 39, 93, 94
state(s), 11, 22, 23, 24, 25, 31, 32, 34, 83, 84, 111
statistics, 74
stenosis, 86
stimulant(s), viii, 65, 89, 91, 110
stimulation, 4, 77, 78
stomach, 48
stratification, 17, 31, 73, 100, 111
stress, 18, 27, 38, 51, 58, 78, 93, 94, 95, 96, 116, 117, 118, 119
stressful life events, 96
stressors, 78
Stunting, 93
style, 62, 63
substitution, 18
succession, 7
sudden cardiac death, 17, 27, 55, 58, 64, 66, 68, 84, 89, 99, 111, 118
sudden death, 6, 65, 89, 119
Sudden infant death syndrome, 64
sudden unexpected death in epilepsy, 49, 99, 101
SUDEP, 100, 101, 111
superior vena cava, 58
supplementation, 34, 36, 40, 41, 42, 45, 62, 64, 65, 107, 118, 119
suppression, 51
supraventricular tachycardia, 69
surface area, 78
surgery of congenital heart defects, 57, 58
survival, 84
survivors, 64, 77, 111, 116
sympathetic denervation, 71, 110
sympathetic nervous system, 26, 56, 109
symptoms, 48, 56, 93, 112
syndrome, 32, 38, 40, 48, 64, 68, 117

## T

tachycardia, 69
tachypnea, 56
target, 49
Task Force, 107
teachers, 13
technical assistance, viii
technology, ix, 19, 43, 106
testing, 21, 78
tetralogy, 62, 63, 86, 87, 110, 111, 114

thalassemia, 113
therapeutic approaches, 32
therapeutic effects, 40
therapy, vii, 11, 34, 37, 45, 46, 47, 49, 55, 58, 62, 63, 64, 69, 73, 74, 75, 82, 83, 84, 86, 88, 96, 97, 100, 105, 106, 115, 117
thin healthy children, 21
thoracic pain, 48
Time Domain Analysis, 1, 3, 7, 9
time frame, x, 1
tobacco, 119
tobacco smoke, 119
tonic, 99
tonic-clonic seizures, 99
Total Power, x, 2, 3, 27, 28, 29, 34, 75
toxin, 43
training, 28, 30, 31, 51, 110, 111
transposition of the great arteries, 58, 111
treatment, 3, 34, 35, 38, 45, 55, 58, 63, 65, 78, 82, 84, 88, 89, 91, 94, 101, 107, 109, 110, 114
trial, 84, 86, 96, 114, 116, 119
Turkey, 5, 17
type 1 diabetes, 112, 117

## U

uniform, 101
United Kingdom (UK), 113, 114
United States, 5, 17, 89
USA, 13, 55

## V

vagal activity, 3, 4, 5, 14, 15, 17, 45, 46, 47, 49, 51, 69, 89, 90, 106
vagal maturation, 14, 16, 69, 106
vagal shift, 5, 15, 17, 106
vagus, 27, 69, 71, 110
validation, 11
valve, 63
vasculature, 119
ventricle, 116
ventricular arrhythmias, 65, 115
ventricular parasystole, 65
ventricular septal defect, 118
ventricular tachycardia, 17, 58, 68
very low frequency, 26, 27
virus infection, 48
visceral adiposity, 117
VSD, 96
vulnerability, 89

## W

weight gain, 32, 33, 35, 36, 37, 96, 113
well-being, 93
withdrawal, 28
wood, 99
workers, 119
worldwide, 17
WPW syndrome, 68

## Y

young adults, 71, 86, 87, 109, 110, 119
young people, 101